Diabetic Cakes, Pies & Other Scrumptious Desserts

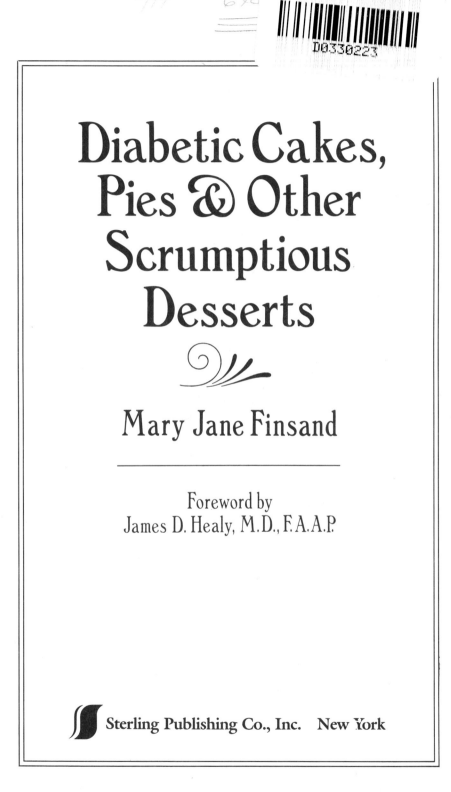

Mary Jane Finsand

Foreword by
James D. Healy, M.D., F.A.A.P.

Sterling Publishing Co., Inc.   New York

EDITED BY LAUREL ORNITZ

RECIPE CONSULTANT: CAROL TIFFANY

Library of Congress Cataloging-in-Publication Data

Finsand, Mary Jane.
   Diabetic cakes, pies, & other scrumptious desserts / Mary Jane
Finsand; foreword by James D. Healy.
   p.   cm.
   Includes index.
   ISBN 0-8069-6673-4   ISBN 0-8069-6672-6 (pbk.)
   1. Diabetes—Diet therapy—Recipes. 2. Desserts. I. Title.
II. Title: Diabetic cakes, pies, and other scrumptious desserts.
RC662.F5626   1988
641.8′6—dc19   87-26749
                                                                                       CIP

Copyright © 1988 by Mary Jane Finsand
Published by Sterling Publishing Co., Inc.
387 Park Avenue South, New York, N.Y. 10016
Distributed in Canada by Sterling Publishing
% Canadian Manda Group, P.O. Box 920, Station U
Toronto, Ontario, Canada M8Z 5P9
Distributed in Great Britain and Europe by Cassell PLC
Artillery House, Artillery Row, London SW1P 1RT, England
Distributed in Australia by Capricorn Ltd.
P.O. Box 665, Lane Cove, NSW 2066
Manufactured in the United States of America
All rights reserved

Contents

Foreword

For many people, the sweet, satisfying taste of dessert is what really makes the meal. However, diabetics and other people concerned about their diets often must skip dessert because sugary foods are so high in calories and carbohydrates.

Mary Jane Finsand has written *Diabetic Cakes, Pies & Other Scrumptious Desserts* for the people who have always had to skip these treats. Each recipe includes calories, carbohydrates, and exchanges, allowing diabetics to regulate their food intake according to their doctor's recommendations. Using these recipes, diabetics and weight watchers will delight in being able to eat sweets again, while still keeping healthy nutritional habits.

Mary Jane's collection of cookbooks is a wonderful series for diet-conscious people. Look for her other diabetic cookbooks—I recommend them all!

James D. Healy, M.D., F.A.A.P.

Preface

Most people think that being on a diet means giving up cakes, pies, tortes, and soufflés. But you can actually eat these foods if you alter their recipes by substituting common table sugar with artificial sugar replacements and super-sweet natural sugars to lower their calories and carbohydrates.

Mary Jane Finsand's *Diabetic Cakes, Pies & Other Scrumptious Desserts* cookbook contains such recipes. Especially intended for diabetics and weight watchers, the recipes are easy to follow, and have exchanges, calories, and carbohydrates listed for each serving.

We recommend *Diabetic Cakes, Pies & Other Scrumptious Desserts* to many of our diet-conscious patients. Other books we recommend include Mary Jane's *Diabetic Breakfast & Brunch Cookbook, Diabetic Gourmet Cookbook, Diabetic Snack & Appetizer Cookbook,* and *Diabetic Chocolate Cookbook.*

Hattie M. Middleton, R.D.
Darlene K. Duke, R.N.
Covenant Medical Center
Waterloo, Iowa

Introduction

With the introduction of sorbitol, fructose, xylitol, and aspartame sweeteners, diabetics and weight watchers can now enjoy better tasting desserts, and thus can add many new exchanges and delicious foods to their diets.

In this book, I have done many of the things you have requested. For example, many of the desserts are made with fructose or sorbitol, or both of them along with an artificial sugar replacement, which gives them the aroma and taste you like. Most of the fillings for the pies are calculated separately from the crust; this allows you to use any crust you want. In addition, there are several recipes that include already prepared products, giving you more time to enjoy other things in life.

However, I must emphasize that you should have desserts in moderation. A dessert is a "fun" food, but make sure that you calculate it as part of your diet. Do not think you can slip it by your normal diet requirements; you cannot.

If you are a diabetic, your diet has probably been prescribed by a doctor or diet counsellor who has determined your diet requirements by considering your exercise and other daily life patterns. Do not try to outguess your doctor or counsellor. Always stay within the guidelines of your individual diet, and be sure to ask about any additions or substitutions. If you have questions about any diabetic recipes or exchanges, ask your doctor or diet counsellor.

I wish to thank my many friends and neighbors who have given of their time and taste buds to make this book possible. I hope this cookbook will help you with your food selections and will help keep you on a balanced diet.

Mary Jane Finsand

Sweeteners

You can find most sweeteners, or sugar replacements, in your local supermarket. They vary in terms of sweetness, aftertaste, aroma, and calories. The listing below is by ingredient name rather than product name. When you are shopping, check the side of the box or bottle to determine the contents of the product.

Aspartame and aspartame products are new additions to the supermarket. Aspartame is a natural protein sweetener. Because of its intense sweetness, it reduces calories and carbohydrates in the diet. Aspartame has a sweet aroma and no aftertaste. However, it does lose some of its sweetness in heating, and is therefore recommended for use in cold products.

Cyclamates and products containing cyclamates are not as sweet as saccharin and saccharin products, and also leave a bitter aftertaste. Many sugar replacements consist of a combination of saccharin and cyclamates.

Fructose is commonly known as fruit sugar. It's actually a natural sugar found in fruits and honey. Fructose tastes the same as common table sugar (sucrose), but because of its intense sweetness, it reduces calories and carbohydrates in the diet. It is not affected by heating or cooling, but baked products made with fructose tend to be heavier.

Glycyrrhizin and products containing glycyrrhizin are as sweet as saccharin and saccharin products. However, they are less available in supermarkets because they give food a licorice taste and aroma.

Saccharin and products containing saccharin are the most widely known and used intense sweeteners. When used in baking or cooking, saccharin has a lingering, bitter aftertaste. You will usually find it in the form of sodium saccharin in products that are labelled low-calorie sugar replacements. Granular or dry sugar replacements containing sodium saccharin give less of an aftertaste to foods that are heated. But it's best to use liquid sugar replacements containing sodium saccharin in cold foods or in foods that have partially cooled and no longer need any heating.

Sorbitol is used in many commercial food products. It has little or no aftertaste and a sweet aroma. At present it can only be bought in bulk form at health-food outlets.

Stevia Rebaudian is a natural sweetener that is not as sweet as saccharin but still a hundred times sweeter than common table sugar. It comes in an herbal form, and can be added directly to the recipe. Or it can be steeped like tea and strained, producing a handy liquid sweetener. But keep in mind that the added liquid will have to be compensated for in the overall ingredients.

Xylitol is a natural sweetener made from birch tree bark. It usually comes in a granular form the same way as sugar, but it's much sweeter. It has no aftertaste, and works well in both hot and cold foods.

If you have difficulty finding these products, you can try contacting a distributor or a mail-order outlet. I have been able to buy the sweeteners in bulk and smaller quantities from these two companies:

NOW Foods
Distributor of Natural Foods Products
721 North Yale
Villa Park, Illinois 60181

The Fruitful Yield
4950 West Oakton
Skokie, Illinois 60077
(312) 679-8975

Using the Recipes – Conversion Guides, Flavorings & Extracts, Spices & Herbs

Read the recipes carefully. Then assemble all equipment and ingredients. Use standard measuring equipment (whether metric or customary), and be sure to measure accurately. Remember, these recipes are good for everyone, not just the diabetic.

Customary Terms

t.	teaspoon	qt.	quart
T.	tablespoon	oz.	ounce
c.	cup	lb.	pound
pkg.	package	°F	degrees Fahrenheit
pt.	pint	in.	inch

Metric Symbols

mL	millilitre	°C	degrees Celsius
L	litre	mm	millimetre
g	gram	cm	centimetre
kg	kilogram		

Conversion Guide for Cooking Pans and Casseroles

Customary	Metric
1 qt.	1 L
2 qt.	2 L
3 qt.	3 L

Oven-Cooking Guides

Fahrenheit °F	Oven Heat	Celsius °C
250–275°	very slow	120–135°
300–325°	slow	150–165°
350–375°	moderate	175–190°
400–425°	hot	200–220°
450–475°	very hot	230–245°
475–500°	hottest	250–290°

Use this candy-thermometer guide to test for doneness:

Fahrenheit °F	Test		Celsius °C
230–234°	Syrup:	Thread	100–112°
234–240°	Fondant/Fudge:	Soft Ball	112–115°
244–248°	Caramels:	Firm Ball	118–120°
250–266°	Marshmallows:	Hard Ball	121–130°
270–290°	Taffy:	Soft Crack	132–143°
300–310°	Brittle:	Hard Crack	149–154°

Guide to Approximate Equivalents

Customary				Metric	
Ounces Pounds	Cups	Tablespoons	Teaspoons	Millilitres	Grams Kilograms
			¼ t.	1 mL	1g
			½ t.	2 mL	
			1 t.	5 mL	
			2 t.	10 mL	
½ oz.		1 T.	3 t.	15 mL	15 g
1 oz.		2 T.	6 t.	30 mL	30 g
2 oz.	¼ c.	4 T.	12 t.	60 mL	
4 oz.	½ c.	8 T.	24 t.	125 mL	
8 oz.	1 c.	16 T.	48 t.	250 mL	
2.2 lb.					1 kg

Keep in mind that this guide does not show exact conversions, but it can be used in a general way for food measurement.

Guide to Baking-Pan Sizes

Customary	Metric	Holds	Holds (Metric)
8-in. pie	20-cm pie	2 c.	600 mL
9-in. pie	23-cm pie	1 qt.	1 L
10-in. pie	25-cm pie	1¼ qt.	1.3 L
8-in. round	20-cm round	1 qt.	1 L
9-in. round	23-cm round	1½ qt.	1.5 L
8-in. square	20-cm square	2 qt.	2 L
9-in. square	23-cm square	2½ qt.	2.5 L
9 × 5 × 2 loaf	23 × 13 × 5 cm (loaf)	2 qt.	2 L
9-in. tube	23-cm tube	3 qt.	3 L
10-in. tube	25-cm tube	3 qt.	3 L
10-in. Bundt	25-cm Bundt	3 qt.	3 L
9 × 5 in.	23 × 13 cm	1½ qt.	1.5 L
10 × 6 in.	25 × 16 cm	3½ qt.	3.5 L
11 × 7 in.	27 × 17 cm	3½ qt.	3.5 L
13 × 9 × 2 in.	33 × 23 × 5 cm	3½ qt.	3.5 L
14 × 10 in.	36 × 25 cm	cookie tin	
15½ × 10½ × 1 in.	39 × 25 × 3 cm	jelly roll	

Flavorings & Extracts

Orange, lime, and lemon peels give pastries and puddings a fresh, clean flavor. Liquor flavors, such as brandy and rum, give cakes and other desserts a company flair. Choose from the following to give your recipes some zip, without adding calories:

Almond	Butter rum	Pecan
Anise (Licorice)	Cherry	Peppermint
Apricot	Chocolate	Pineapple
Banana creme	Coconut	Raspberry
Blackberry	Grape	Rum
Black walnut	Hazelnut	Sassafras
Blueberry	Lemon	Sherry
Brandy	Lime	Strawberry
Butter	Mint	Vanilla
Butternut	Orange	Walnut

Spices & Herbs

This is a summary of some of my favorite spices and herbs. They will definitely add distinction to your desserts, without adding calories.

Allspice: cinnamon, ginger, and nutmeg flavor; used in breads, pastries, jellies, jams, and pickles.

Anise: licorice flavor; used in candies, breads, fruit, wine, and liqueurs.

Cinnamon: pungent, sweet flavor; used in pastries, breads, pickles, wine, beer, and liqueurs.

Clove: pungent, sweet flavor; used in ham, sauces, pastries, puddings, fruit, wine, and liqueurs.

Coriander: bitter-lemon flavor; used in cookies, cakes, pies, puddings, fruit, and wine and liqueur punches.

Ginger: strong, pungent flavor; used in anything sweet, also with beer, brandy, and liqueurs.

Nutmeg: sweet, nutty flavor; used in pastries, puddings, and vegetables.

Woodruff: sweet, vanilla flavor; used in wines and punches.

Cakes

White Cake

1½ c.	cake flour	375 mL
1½ t.	baking powder	7 mL
¼ t.	salt	1 mL
¼ c.	solid shortening	60 mL
½ c.	sorbitol	125 mL
2 t.	clear vanilla flavoring	10 mL
1 t.	water	5 mL
½ c.	2 % low-fat milk	125 mL
2	egg whites, stiffly beaten	2

Combine cake flour, baking powder, and salt in a sifter, and then sift into a medium-size bowl. Set aside. Beat shortening, sorbitol, vanilla, and water together until creamy. Add flour mixture and milk alternately, beating well after each addition. Fold in stiffly beaten egg whites. Grease an 8-in. (20-cm) cake pan. Line pan with waxed paper and grease it again; then flour pan lightly. Spread batter into greased, lined, and floured cake pan. Bake at 350 °F (175 °C) for 30 to 35 minutes or until toothpick inserted in center comes out clean. Allow to cool. Turn over onto board or plate, and remove waxed paper.

Yield: 10 servings
Exchange, 1 serving: 1 starch/bread, 1 fat
Calories, 1 serving: 105
Carbohydrates, 1 serving: 12

White Angel-Food Cake

1 c.	sifted cake flour	250 mL
1 c.	sorbitol	250 mL
10	egg whites	10
1 t.	cream of tartar	5 mL
½ t.	salt	2 mL
1 t.	vanilla extract	5 mL
½ t.	almond extract	2 mL

Sift cake flour three times. Blend sorbitol on HIGH in blender until mixture becomes a fine powder. Stir ¼ c. (60 mL) of sorbitol powder into flour. Now beat egg whites, cream of tartar, and salt together until frothy. Add remaining sorbitol in small amounts to egg whites, beating well after each addition. Continue beating until mixture will hold stiff peaks. Beat in extracts. Sift one-fourth of the flour mixture over the egg whites; then gently fold it in. Continue in this manner with the remaining flour mixture, adding one-fourth at a time. Pour the batter into a 10-in. (25-cm) ungreased tube pan. Bake at 350 °F (175 °C) for 50 to 60 minutes or until done. Invert and cool completely. Remove cake from pan.

Yield: 20 servings
Exchange, 1 serving: ½ starch/bread
Calories, 1 serving: 40
Carbohydrates, 1 serving: 5

Pastry White Cake

4 c.	cake flour	1000 mL
4 t.	baking powder	20 mL
½ t.	salt	2 mL
1 c.	solid shortening	250 mL
1 T.	almond extract	15 mL
1 T.	warm water	15 mL
1 t.	vanilla extract	5 mL
1½ c.	sorbitol	375 mL
½ c.	granulated sugar replacement	125 mL
1 c.	skim milk	250 mL
10	egg whites, stiffly beaten	10

Combine cake flour, baking powder, and salt in a sifter, and sift into a bowl. Set aside. Beat shortening, almond extract, water, and vanilla together until creamy. Add sorbitol and granulated sugar replacement.

Beat until fluffy. Add flour mixture and milk alternately in small amounts, beating well after each addition. Fold in stiffly beaten egg whites. Grease a 15½ × 10½ × 1 in. (39 × 25 × 3 cm) jelly-roll pan. Line bottom of pan with waxed paper and grease again. Flour lightly. Spread batter into greased, lined, and floured pan. Bake at 350 °F (175 °C) for 25 to 30 minutes or until toothpick inserted in center comes out clean. Allow to cool. Carefully turn over onto a cutting board. Remove waxed paper. Cut into 50 pieces — you might want to try oblongs, squares, circles, and diamonds, or even more unusual shapes.

Yield: 50 servings
Exchange, 1 serving: ¾ starch/bread, ¾ fat
Calories, 1 serving: 95
Carbohydrates, 1 serving: 12

Party White Cake

3 c.	cake flour	750 mL
3 t.	baking powder	15 mL
½ t.	salt	2 mL
¾ c.	solid shortening	190 mL
1½ c.	granulated sugar replacement	375 mL
3 T.	water	45 mL
½ c.	skim milk	125 mL
½ c.	warm water	125 mL
2 t.	vanilla extract	10 mL
6	egg whites, stiffly beaten	6

Combine cake flour, baking powder, and salt in a sifter. Sift into a large bowl. Set aside. Cream shortening, granulated sugar replacement, and 3-T. (45-mL) water together until fluffy. Combine milk, ½ c. (125-mL) warm water, and vanilla in a measuring cup. Add sifted ingredients and liquid ingredients alternately in small amounts to creamed shortening, beating well after each addition. Fold cake batter into egg whites. Pour into three 9-in. (23-cm) greased and floured cake pans. Bake at 350 °F (175 °C) for 25 to 30 minutes or until toothpick inserted in center comes out clean. Allow to cool slightly in pans. Then remove from pans and allow to cool completely on racks.

Yield: 20 servings
Exchange, 1 serving: 1 starch/bread, 1 fat
Calories, 1 serving: 121
Carbohydrates, 1 serving: 15

Banana Spice Cake

2¾ c.	sifted all-purpose flour	690 mL
2 t.	baking powder	10 mL
1 t.	baking soda	5 mL
1 t.	salt	5 mL
2 t.	cinnamon	10 mL
1 t.	nutmeg	5 mL
¼ t.	cloves	1 mL
⅔ c.	solid shortening	180 mL
1 c.	granulated sugar replacement	250 mL
2 T.	water	30 mL
1 t.	vinegar	5 mL
2	eggs, well beaten	2
1½ c.	mashed bananas	375 mL
2 t.	vanilla extract	10 mL

Sift flour, baking powder, baking soda, salt, and spices together three times. Set aside. Beat shortening, sugar replacement, water, and vinegar together until fluffy. Add eggs and beat well. Add sifted ingredients and mashed bananas alternately in small amounts to creamed mixture, beating well after each addition. Stir in vanilla. Transfer to greased and floured 13×9 in. (33×23 cm) cake pan. Bake at 350 °F (175 °C) for 35 to 45 minutes or until toothpick inserted in center comes out clean.

Yield: 24 servings
Exchange, 1 serving: 1½ starch/bread, ⅔ fat, ⅓ fruit
Calories, 1 serving: 130
Carbohydrates, 1 serving: 23

Orange Rum Cake

1 c.	warm buttermilk	250 mL
2 t.	Stevia Rebaudian Herb	10 mL
1 c.	low-calorie margarine	250 mL
2 T.	grated fresh orange rind	30 mL
2	eggs	2
2½ c.	sifted all-purpose flour	625 mL
2 t.	baking powder	10 mL
1 t.	baking soda	5 mL
½ t.	salt	2 mL
½ c.	orange juice	125 mL

| 1 T. | lemon juice | 15 mL |
| 2 T. | rum | 30 mL |

Combine warm buttermilk and Stevia Rebaudian, stirring to blend. Allow to sweeten for 2 hours. Beat margarine until creamy. Beat in orange rind. Then beat in eggs, one at a time (beating well after each addition). Combine flour, baking powder, baking soda, and salt in a sifter. Sift into a bowl. Add sifted ingredients and sweetened buttermilk alternately in small amounts to creamed mixture, beating until very smooth. Pour batter into a well greased 10-in. (25-cm) tube pan. Bake at 350 °F (175 °C) for 60 to 70 minutes or until cake tester inserted in center comes out clean. Now combine juices and rum in a small saucepan. Heat to boiling. When cake is done, remove from oven. Slowly pour hot juice mixture over cake in pan. Allow cake to cool; then wrap and refrigerate for 1 or 2 days before serving.

Yield: 30 servings
Exchange, 1 serving: ¾ starch/bread, 1 fat
Calories, 1 serving: 104
Carbohydrates, 1 serving: 13

Almond-Flavored Cake

18	eggs	18
¾ c.	granulated fructose	190 mL
1 t.	vanilla extract	5 mL
½ t.	almond extract	2 mL
2 c.	sifted cake flour	500 mL
¼ c.	butter, melted	60 mL

Combine eggs and fructose in top of double boiler. Beat to blend. Place over simmering water. (Do not allow water to boil!) Continue beating for about 10 or 12 minutes or until very light and fluffy. Remove from heat, and then beat until cool. Beat in vanilla and almond extracts. Fold in cake flour very gradually. Add melted butter and fold well. (Do not stir.) Pour batter into three 9-in. (23-cm) round greased cake pans. Bake at 325 °F (165 °C) for 30 to 35 minutes or until done. Remove from oven. Remove cakes from pans, and cool completely on racks.

Yield: 30 servings
Exchange, 1 serving: ½ starch/bread, ½ fat, ½ high-fat meat
Calories, 1 serving: 102
Carbohydrates, 1 serving: 7

Apple Walnut Cake

1 qt.	chopped apples	1 L
¼ c.	granulated fructose	60 mL
½ c.	granulated sugar replacement	125 mL
1 t.	lemon juice	5 mL
2 c.	sifted all-purpose flour	500 mL
2 t.	baking soda	10 mL
2 t.	cinnamon	10 mL
1 t.	salt	5 mL
½ c.	liquid shortening	125 mL
2	eggs, well beaten	2
2 t.	vanilla extract	10 mL
½ c.	chopped walnuts	125 mL

Combine chopped apples, fructose, sugar replacement, and lemon juice in a bowl. Toss to coat apples. Set aside for 15 minutes. Sift flour, baking soda, cinnamon, and salt together three times. Beat liquid shortening and eggs together until well mixed. Beat in vanilla. Add sifted ingredients and beat until blended. Add apple mixture and stir very well for at least 2 minutes. Fold in walnuts. Transfer to greased and floured 13×9 in. (33×23 cm) cake pan. Bake at 350 °F (175 °C) for 55 to 60 minutes or until toothpick inserted in center comes out clean.

Yield: 24 servings
Exchange, 1 serving: 1 starch/bread, ⅓ fat
Calories, 1 serving: 86
Carbohydrates, 1 serving: 13

Real Sponge Cake

1 c.	sifted cake flour	250 mL
¼ t.	salt	1 mL
1 T.	grated fresh lemon rind	15 mL
1½ T.	fresh lemon juice	21 mL
5	eggs, separated	5
½ c.	sorbitol	125 mL

Sift cake flour and salt together four times. Set aside. Add lemon rind and lemon juice to egg yolks. Beat until very thick. Beat egg whites until very stiff peaks form. Fold sorbitol into egg whites. Then fold in egg-yolk mixture. Sift the flour mixture, a fourth of it at a time, over the top of the egg mixture. Gently fold the flour in after each addition. Pour into a 9-in. (23-cm) ungreased tube pan. Bake at 350 °F (175 °C) for 60 minutes or until done. Invert pan and cool completely. Remove cake from pan.

Yield: 20 servings
Exchange, 1 serving: ¾ starch/bread, ⅓ fat
Calories, 1 serving: 83
Carbohydrates, 1 serving: 11

Apple Upside-Down Cake

2 T.	low-calorie margarine	30 mL
½ c.	dietetic maple syrup	125 mL
2 large	baking apples	2 large
¼ c.	raisins	60 mL
1½ c.	sifted cake flour	375 mL
3 t.	baking soda	15 mL
½ t.	salt	2 mL
⅓ c.	solid shortening	90 mL
⅓ c.	granulated sugar replacement	90 mL
1 T.	water	15 mL
2	eggs, well beaten	2
1 t.	vanilla extract	5 mL
⅔ c.	water	180 mL

Melt low-calorie margarine in bottom of 9-in. (23-cm) cake pan. Add maple syrup, stirring to mix. Allow to cool. Peel, core, and slice apples; then layer over margarine-syrup mixture in cake pan. Sprinkle with raisins. Combine cake flour, baking soda, and salt in sifter, and sift into bowl. Cream together shortening, sugar replacement and 1-T. (15-mL) water. Beat in eggs and vanilla. Add sifted ingredients and ⅔-c. (180-mL) water alternately in small amounts, beating well after each addition. Pour over apples in pan. Lightly spread to level the batter. Bake at 350 °F (175 °C) for 45 to 50 minutes or until toothpick inserted in center comes out clean. Turn over onto a serving plate immediately after removing from oven.

Yield: 24 servings
Exchange, 1 serving: ⅔ starch/bread, ⅓ fat, ¼ fruit
Calories, 1 serving: 90
Carbohydrates, 1 serving: 11

Pineapple Chiffon Cake

2¼ c.	sifted cake flour	560 mL
1 T.	baking powder	15 mL
½ t.	salt	2 mL
¾ c.	sorbitol	190 mL
½ c.	liquid vegetable oil	125 mL
5	egg yolks	5
¾ c.	unsweetened pineapple juice	190 mL
8	egg whites	8
¾ t.	cream of tartar	4 mL

Combine cake flour, baking powder, and salt in a sifter. Sift into a large mixing bowl. Add sorbitol. Make a well in the center of flour mixture, and add vegetable oil, egg yolks, and pineapple juice. Beat until mixture becomes very smooth and thick. Now beat egg whites with cream of tartar into very stiff peaks. Pour batter over egg whites in a thin stream. Fold batter gently into egg whites. Transfer to ungreased 10-in. (25-cm) tube pan. Bake at 350 °F (175 °C) for an hour or until cake tests done. Invert and cool completely. Cut around sides and tube stem. Remove bottom of pan with cake. Carefully cut between cake and pan bottom. Remove cake.

Yield: 24 servings
Exchange, 1 serving: 1 starch/bread, 1 fat
Calories, 1 serving: 102
Carbohydrates, 1 serving: 14

Orange-Sunrise Chiffon Cake

7	egg yolks	7
½ c.	sorbitol	125 mL
2 t.	grated fresh orange rind	10 mL
⅓ c.	orange juice	90 mL
1 c.	sifted cake flour	250 mL
7	egg whites	7
1 t.	cream of tartar	5 mL

Beat egg yolks until they become very thick and lemon colored. Beat in ¼ c. (60 mL) of the sorbitol. Beat in orange rind. Add orange juice and cake flour alternately in small amounts to egg-yolk mixture, beating until mixture becomes very smooth and thick. Now beat egg whites and cream of tartar together until soft peaks form. Beat in remaining ¼ c. (60 mL) of the sorbitol. Beat into very firm peaks. Fold egg whites into batter. Pour into 9-in. (23-cm) ungreased tube pan. Bake at 350 °F (175 °C) for 50 to 60 minutes or until done. Invert and cool completely. Remove cake from pan.

Yield: 24 servings
Exchange, 1 serving: ½ starch/bread
Calories, 1 serving: 41
Carbohydrates, 1 serving: 7

Chocolate Chiffon Cake

4 sq. (1 oz. each)	unsweetened chocolate, melted	4 sq. (30 g each)
½ c.	boiling water	125 mL
¼ c.	granulated fructose	60 mL
2¼ c.	sifted cake flour	560 mL
¾ c.	sorbitol	190 mL
¼ c.	granulated sugar replacement	60 mL
1 T.	baking powder	15 mL
1 t.	salt	5 mL
½ c.	liquid vegetable oil	125 mL
7	egg yolks	7
¾ c.	cold water	190 mL
1½ T.	vanilla extract	21 mL
7	egg whites	7 mL
½ t.	cream of tartar	2 mL

Blend together melted chocolate, boiling water, and fructose. Allow to cool completely. Sift together cake flour, sorbitol, sugar replacement, baking powder, and salt into a large bowl. Make a well in the center of the flour mixture, and add vegetable oil, egg yolks, cold water, and vanilla. Beat until mixture becomes very smooth and thick. Stir cooled chocolate into mixture. Now beat egg whites and cream of tartar into very stiff peaks. Pour batter over egg whites in a thin stream. Fold batter gently into egg whites. Transfer to ungreased 10-in. (25-cm) tube pan. Bake at 325 °F (165 °C) for an hour or until cake tests done. Invert and cool completely. Cut around sides and tube stem. Remove bottom of pan with cake. Carefully cut between cake and pan bottom. Remove cake.

Yield: 30 servings
Exchange, 1 serving: 1 starch/bread, 1⅓ fat
Calories, 1 serving: 123
Carbohydrates, 1 serving: 18

Coffee Chiffon Cake

4 t.	instant coffee, powder	20 mL
¾ c.	boiling water	190 mL
2¼ c.	sifted cake flour	560 mL
1 c.	sorbitol	250 mL
¼ c.	granulated sugar replacement	60 mL
1 T.	baking powder	15 mL
1 t.	salt	5 mL
½ c.	liquid vegetable oil	125 mL
5	egg yolks	5
1 t.	vanilla extract	5 mL
2 sq. (1 oz. each)	semi-sweet chocolate, grated	2 sq. (30 g each)
7	egg whites	7 mL
½ t.	cream of tartar	2 mL

Dissolve coffee powder in boiling water. Cool completely. Sift together cake flour, sorbitol, sugar replacement, baking powder, and salt into a large bowl. Make a well in the center of the flour mixture, and add vegetable oil, egg yolks, and vanilla. Beat until mixture becomes very smooth and thick. Stir in grated chocolate. Now beat egg whites and cream of tartar together into very stiff peaks. Pour batter over egg whites in a thin stream. Fold batter gently into egg whites. Transfer to ungreased 10-in. (25-cm) tube pan. Bake at 325 °F (165 °C) for 70 minutes or until cake tests done. Invert and cool completely. Cut around sides and tube stem. Remove bottom of pan with cake. Carefully cut between cake and pan bottom. Remove cake.

Yield: 20 servings
Exchange, 1 serving: 1 starch/bread, 1 fat
Calories, 1 serving: 119
Carbohydrates, 1 serving: 17

Vanilla Chiffon Cake

2¼ c.	sifted cake flour	560 mL
1 T.	baking powder	15 mL
1 t.	salt	5 mL
1 c.	sorbitol	250 mL
½ c.	liquid vegetable oil	125 mL
8	egg yolks	8
¾ c.	water	190 mL
2 T.	vanilla extract	30 mL

½ t.	lemon juice	2 mL
8	egg whites	8
½ t.	cream of tartar	2 mL

Combine cake flour, baking powder, and salt in a sifter. Sift into a large mixing bowl. Stir in sorbitol. Make a well in the center of the flour mixture, and add vegetable oil, egg yolks, water, vanilla, and lemon juice. Beat until mixture becomes very smooth and thick. Now beat egg whites and cream of tartar together until very stiff peaks form. Fold egg whites into batter. Transfer to 10-in. (25-cm) ungreased tube pan. Bake at 325 °F (165 °C) for 55 to 60 minutes or until done. Invert and cool completely. Remove from pan.

Yield: 24 servings
Exchange, 1 serving: 1 starch/bread, ⅓ fat
Calories, 1 serving: 79
Carbohydrates, 1 serving: 11

Best Lemon Chiffon Cake

8	egg yolks	8
⅔ c.	granulated sorbitol	90 mL
2 t.	grated fresh lemon rind	10 mL
2 t.	unsweetened lemon-drink mix	10 mL
⅓ c.	water	90 mL
1 c.	sifted cake flour	250 mL
8	egg whites	8
1 t.	cream of tartar	5 mL

Beat egg yolks until they become very thick and lemon colored. Beat in ⅓ c. (45 mL) of the sorbitol. Beat in lemon rind and lemon-drink mix. Add water and cake flour alternately in small amounts to egg-yolk mixture, beating until mixture becomes very smooth and thick. Now beat egg whites and cream of tartar together until soft peaks form. Beat in remaining ⅓ c. (45 mL) of the sorbitol. Beat into very firm peaks. Fold egg whites into batter. Pour into 9-in. (23-cm) ungreased tube pan. Bake at 325 °F (165 °C) for 60 to 65 minutes or until done. Invert and cool completely. Remove cake from pan.

Yield: 20 servings
Exchange, 1 serving: ½ starch/bread
Calories, 1 serving: 43
Carbohydrates, 1 serving: 7

Maple Walnut Chiffon Cake

2¼ c.	sifted cake flour	560 mL
3 t.	baking powder	15 mL
1 t.	salt	5 mL
⅔ c.	granulated fructose	180 mL
½ c.	granulated brown-sugar replacement	125 mL
½ c.	liquid vegetable oil	125 mL
5	egg yolks	5
1 T.	maple flavoring	15 mL
¾ c.	cold water	190 mL
9	egg whites	9
1 t.	cream of tartar	5 mL
½ c.	finely chopped walnuts	125 mL

Combine cake flour, baking powder, and salt in a sifter. Sift into a large bowl. Add fructose and stir. Make a well in the flour mixture, and add brown-sugar replacement, vegetable oil, egg yolks, maple flavoring, and water. Beat until mixture becomes very smooth and thick. Now beat egg whites and cream of tartar together until very stiff peaks form. Pour batter in a thin stream over egg whites. Fold gently. Then fold in nuts. Transfer to 10-in. (25-cm) ungreased tube pan. Bake at 350 °F (175 °C) for 60 minutes or until cake tests done. Invert until completely cooled. Remove from pan.

Yield: 30 servings
Exchange, 1 serving: ¾ starch/bread, 1⅓ fat
Calories, 1 serving: 128
Carbohydrates, 1 serving: 12

South Seas Chiffon Cake

2¼ c.	sifted cake flour	560 mL
1 T.	baking powder	15 mL
1 t.	salt	5 mL
1 c.	sorbitol	250 mL
½ c.	granulated sugar replacement	125 mL
½ c.	liquid vegetable oil	125 mL
8	egg yolks	8
1 t.	grated lemon peel	5 mL
1 t.	grated orange peel	5 mL
1 t.	grated lime peel	5 mL
½ c.	orange juice	125 mL

1 T.	lemon juice	15 mL
1 T.	lime juice	15 mL
8	egg whites	8
½ t.	cream of tartar	2 mL

Combine cake flour, baking powder, and salt in a sifter. Sift into a large mixing bowl. Stir in sorbitol and sugar replacement. Make a well in the center of the flour mixture, and add vegetable oil, egg yolks, grated fruit peels, and fruit juices. Beat until mixture becomes very smooth and thick. Now beat egg whites and cream of tartar together until very stiff peaks form. Fold egg whites into batter. Transfer to 10-in. (25-cm) ungreased tube pan. Bake at 325 °F (165 °C) for 55 to 60 minutes or until done. Invert and cool completely. Remove from pan.

Yield: 24 servings
Exchange, 1 serving: 1 starch/bread, ⅓ fat
Calories, 1 serving: 82
Carbohydrates, 1 serving: 13

Banana Poppy-Seed Yolk Cake ✓

3 c.	sifted all-purpose flour	750 mL
1 T.	baking powder	15 mL
1 t.	salt	5 mL
1 t.	banana flavoring	5 mL
12	egg yolks	12
1 c.	mashed bananas	250 mL
¼ c.	hot water	60 mL
1 c.	sorbitol	250 mL
¼ c.	poppy seeds	60 mL

Sift flour and baking powder together four times. Set aside. Add salt and banana flavoring to egg yolks. Beat until very thick. Combine mashed bananas and hot water, stirring to blend. Add sorbitol and bananas alternately in small amounts, to egg-yolk mixture, beating until thick after each addition. Fold in poppy seeds. Fold flour mixture, a fourth of it at a time, into batter. Pour into ungreased 10-in. (25-cm) tube pan. Bake at 350 °F (175 °C) for 60 to 65 minutes or until done. Invert and cool completely. Remove from pan.

Yield: 30 servings
Exchange, 1 serving: 1 starch/bread, ⅓ medium-fat meat
Calories, 1 serving: 105
Carbohydrates, 1 serving: 18

Chocolate Chocolate-Chip Cake

3 sq. (1 oz. each)	unsweetened chocolate, melted	3 sq. (30 g. each)
½ c.	boiling water	125 mL
¼ c.	granulated fructose	60 mL
2¼ c.	sifted cake flour	560 mL
¾ c.	sorbitol	190 mL
½ c.	granulated sugar replacement	125 mL
1 T.	baking powder	15 mL
1 t.	salt	5 mL
½ c.	liquid vegetable oil	125 mL
9	egg yolks	9
¾ c.	cold water	190 mL
1½ T.	vanilla extract	21 mL
9	egg whites	9 mL
½ t.	cream of tartar	2 mL
½ c.	mini-chocolate chips	125 mL

Blend together melted chocolate, boiling water, and fructose. Cool completely. Sift together cake flour, sorbitol, sugar replacement, baking powder, and salt into a large bowl. Make a well in the center of the flour mixture, and add vegetable oil, egg yolks, cold water, and vanilla. Beat until mixture becomes very smooth and thick. Stir in cooled chocolate. Now beat egg whites and cream of tartar together into very stiff peaks. Gently fold egg whites into batter. Then fold in chocolate chips. Transfer to ungreased 10-in. (25-cm) tube pan. Bake at 325 °F (165 °C) for 60 to 70 minutes or until cake tests done. Invert and cool completely. Cut around sides and tube stem. Remove bottom of pan with cake. Carefully cut between cake and pan bottom. Remove cake.

Yield: 30 servings
Exchange, 1 serving: 1 starch/bread, 1⅓ fat
Calories, 1 serving: 109
Carbohydrates, 1 serving: 16

Orange Sponge Cake

2 c.	sifted cake flour	500 mL
2 t.	baking powder	10 mL
¼ t.	salt	1 mL
5	egg yolks	5

1⅔ c.	granulated sugar replacement	440 mL
¾ c.	water	190 mL
1½ T.	grated orange rind	21 mL
½ c.	orange juice	125 mL
4	egg whites	4

Sift cake flour, baking powder, and salt together four times. Beat egg yolks and sugar replacement together until thick enough to hold a soft peak. Add water gradually, beating very thoroughly. Combine orange rind and orange juice. Fold in sifted dry ingredients and orange juice alternately in small amounts to the egg-yolk mixture. Now beat the egg whites until very stiff peaks form. Fold egg whites into batter. Pour batter into a 10-in. (25-cm) ungreased tube pan. Bake at 350 °F (175 °C) for 50 to 60 minutes or until done. Invert and cool completely. Remove from pan.

Yield: 20 servings
Exchange, 1 serving: ¾ starch/bread, ⅓ fat
Calories, 1 serving: 84
Carbohydrates, 1 serving: 11

Rainbow Cake

1 recipe	Light White Cake	1 recipe
⅓ c.	raspberries	90 mL
	red food coloring	
⅓ c.	blueberries	90 mL

Follow the recipe for Light White Cake on page 30, but before folding in egg whites, divide batter into three parts. Leave one part plain. Add raspberries and red food coloring to another part, beating to blend. Add blueberries to third part, beating to blend. Divide egg whites evenly between the three batters. Fold in thoroughly. Pour each cake part into a 9-in. (23-cm) cake pan. Pans should be greased and their bottoms lined with greased waxed paper. Bake at 375 °F (190 °C) for 25 to 30 minutes or until done. Cool in pans for 5 minutes. Transfer to racks, peel off paper, and cool completely. Frost as desired.

Yield: 30 servings
Exchange, 1 serving: 1 starch/bread, 1 fat
Calories, 1 serving: 111
Carbohydrates, 1 serving: 13

Chocolate Angel Cake

¾ c.	sifted cake flour	190 mL
¼ c.	cocoa powder	60 mL
1¼ c.	sorbitol	310 mL
12	egg whites	12
1 t.	cream of tartar	5 mL
½ t.	salt	2 mL
1 t.	vanilla extract	5 mL

Sift cake flour and cocoa together four times. Blend sorbitol on HIGH in blender until mixture becomes a fine powder. Stir ¼ c. (60 mL) of the sorbitol powder into the flour-cocoa mixture. Now beat egg whites, cream of tartar, and salt together until frothy. Add remaining sorbitol, in small amounts, to egg whites. Beat well after each addition. Continue beating until mixture will hold stiff peaks. Beat in vanilla. Sift one-fourth of the flour-cocoa mixture over the egg whites; then fold it in lightly. Continue in this manner with the remaining flour-cocoa mixture, adding one-fourth at a time. Pour the batter into a 10-in. (25-cm) ungreased tube pan. Bake at 350 °F (175 °C) for 50 to 60 minutes or until done. Invert and cool completely. Remove cake from pan.

Yield: 20 servings
Exchange, 1 serving: ¾ starch/flour
Calories, 1 serving: 60
Carbohydrates, 1 serving: 9

Toasted-Coconut Angel Cake

½ c.	unsweetened shredded coconut	125 mL
¾ c.	sifted cake flour	190 mL
¾ c.	sorbitol	190 mL
2 T.	granulated sugar replacement	30 mL
10	egg whites	10
1 t.	cream of tartar	5 mL
½ t.	salt	2 mL
1 t.	vanilla extract	5 mL
½ t.	coconut flavoring	2 mL

Place coconut in a small skillet. Lightly brown over low heat. Allow to cool. Pour into blender and blend into a powder. Sift cake flour three times. Stir coconut powder into flour. Blend sorbitol on HIGH in blender until mixture becomes a fine powder. Stir sugar replacement into sorbitol powder, creating a sweetener. Stir ¼ c. (60 mL) of the sweetener into flour-coconut mixture. Now beat egg whites, cream of tartar, and salt together until frothy. Add remaining sweetener in small amounts to egg whites, beating well after each addition. Continue beating until mixture will hold stiff peaks. Beat in vanilla and coconut flavoring. Sift one-fourth of the flour-coconut mixture over the egg whites; then lightly fold it in. Continue in this manner with the remaining flour-coconut mixture, adding one-fourth at a time. Pour the batter into a 10-in. (25-cm) ungreased tube pan. Bake at 350 °F (175 °C) for 50 to 60 minutes or until done. Invert and cool completely. Remove cake from pan.

Yield: 20 servings
Exchange, 1 serving: ½ starch/bread
Calories, 1 serving: 42
Carbohydrates, 1 serving: 7

Chocolate-Chip Angel Cake

1 c.	sifted cake flour	250 mL
1 c.	sorbitol	250 mL
10	egg whites	10
1 t.	cream of tartar	5 mL
½ t.	salt	2 mL
1 t.	vanilla extract	5 mL
½ c.	mini-chocolate chips	125 mL

Sift cake flour three times. Blend sorbitol on HIGH in blender until mixture becomes a fine powder. Stir ¼ c. (60 mL) of the sorbitol powder into the flour. Now beat egg whites, cream of tartar, and salt together until frothy. Add remaining sorbitol in small amounts to egg whites, beating well after each addition. Continue beating until mixture will hold stiff peaks. Beat in vanilla. Sift one-fourth of the flour mixture over the egg whites; then lightly fold it in. Repeat this procedure with the remaining flour mixture, adding one-fourth at a time. Then gently fold in the chocolate chips. (If chips are too large, cut them or process them in a blender.) Pour the batter into a 10-in. (25-cm) ungreased tube pan. Bake at 350 °F (175 °C) for 50 to 60 minutes or until done. Invert and cool completely. Remove cake from pan.

Yield: 20 servings
Exchange, 1 serving: ¾ starch/bread
Calories, 1 serving: 64
Carbohydrates, 1 serving: 12

Light White Cake

⅔ c.	soft butter	180 mL
¾ c.	sorbitol	190 mL
1½ t.	clear vanilla flavoring	7 mL
½ t.	almond extract	2 mL
2½ c.	sifted cake flour	625 mL
2½ t.	baking powder	12 mL
⅔ c.	skim milk	180 mL
4	egg whites	4
½ t.	salt	2 mL
½ t.	cream of tartar	2 mL

Cream butter until light and fluffy. Add sorbitol gradually, beating constantly. Continue beating until mixture is light and fluffy. Beat in vanilla flavoring and almond extract. Combine cake flour and baking powder in sifter. Sift a fourth of the flour mixture over the creamed butter, and then beat thoroughly. Add a third of the skim milk, and then beat thoroughly. Add flour mixture and milk alternately, as stated above, beating thoroughly after each addition. Now beat egg whites until frothy. Add salt and cream of tartar. Beat until stiff peaks form. Fold egg whites into batter. Pour batter into two 9-in. (23-cm) pans. Each pan should be greased and lined on the bottom with greased waxed paper. Bake at 375 °F (190 °C) for 25 to 30 minutes or until done. Cool in pans for 5 minutes. Transfer to racks, peel off paper, and cool completely.

Yield: 30 servings
Exchange, 1 serving: 1 starch/bread, 1 fat
Calories, 1 serving: 110
Carbohydrates, 1 serving: 13

Cream-Filled Chocolate Cake

Cake

¼ c.	granulated sugar replacement	60 mL
3 T.	water	45 mL
2 sq. (1 oz. each)	unsweetened chocolate, melted	2 sq. (30 g each)
¾ c.	low-calorie margarine	190 mL
½ c.	granulated fructose	125 mL
1 c.	granulated sugar replacement	250 mL

1 t.	vanilla extract	5 mL
4	egg yolks	4
2¼ c.	sifted cake flour	560 mL
1 t.	cream of tartar	5 mL
½ t.	baking soda	2 mL
½ t.	salt	2 mL
1 c.	skim milk	250 mL
4	egg whites, stiffly beaten	4

Combine the ¼-c. (60-mL) sugar replacement and water. Add to melted chocolate and stir to blend. Set aside. Cream margarine. Gradually add the fructose and the 1-c. (250-mL) sugar replacement. Beat until light and fluffy. Add vanilla. Add egg yolks, one at a time, beating well after each addition. Beat in chocolate mixture. Sift dry ingredients together, and add to batter alternately with skim milk. (Begin and end with dry ingredients.) Beat until smooth. Fold stiffly beaten egg whites into batter. Pour batter into three 9-in. (23-cm) round pans. Pans should be greased and their bottoms lined with greased waxed paper. Bake at 350 °F (175 °C) for 45 to 50 minutes or until done. Cool in pans for 5 minutes. Transfer to racks, peel off paper and cool completely. Put layers together with Cream Filling.

Cream Filling

¼ c.	granulated fructose	60 mL
3 T.	all-purpose flour	45 mL
dash	salt	dash
1½ c.	skim milk	375 mL
2	eggs, beaten	2
½ t.	vanilla extract	2

In the top of a double boiler, mix fructose, flour, and salt. Add ½ c. (125 mL) of the skim milk. Stir until smooth. Stir in remaining milk. Cook mixture over boiling water, stirring constantly, until thick and smooth. Add small amount of hot mixture to beaten eggs. Stir to blend. Return to top of double boiler. Cook and stir about 5 minutes longer or until mixture is very thick. Allow to cool; then stir in vanilla. Use to fill and lightly frost cooled cake.

Yield: 30 servings
Exchange, 1 serving: 1 starch/bread, ¼ fat
Calories, 1 serving: 99
Carbohydrates, 1 serving: 16

Crumb Cake

2½ c.	sifted cake flour	625 mL
1½ c.	brown-sugar replacement	375 mL
½ c.	solid shortening	125 mL
1	egg, well beaten	1
2 t.	baking powder	10 mL
1½ t.	cinnamon	7 mL
¾ c.	skim milk	190 mL

Combine 2 c. (500 mL) of the sifted cake flour, brown-sugar replacement, and shortening in a bowl or food processor. Cut until mixture is crumbly. Remove ½ c. (125 mL) of the mixture and reserve. Add egg, baking powder, cinnamon, and skim milk to the remainder of the mixture. Mix thoroughly. Spread on bottom of greased and floured 8-in. (20-cm)-square cake pan. Sprinkle with reserved crumbs. Bake at 350 °F (175 °C) for 30 to 40 minutes or until toothpick inserted in center comes out clean.

Yield: 16 servings
Exchange, 1 serving: 1 starch/bread, 1 fat
Calories, 1 serving: 117
Carbohydrates, 1 serving: 13

Magic Devil's Food Cake

5 T.	cocoa powder	75 mL
1	egg yolk	1
1½ c.	skim milk	375 mL
½ c.	low-calorie margarine	125 mL
¾ c.	sorbitol	190 mL
½ c.	granulated sugar replacement	125 mL
1 t.	vanilla extract	5 mL
2	eggs	2
2 c.	sifted all-purpose flour	500 mL
2 t.	baking powder	10 mL
¼ t.	baking soda	1 mL
½ t.	salt	2 mL

Mix cocoa, egg yolk, and 1 c. (250 mL) of the skim milk in a saucepan. Cook over low heat, stirring, until smooth and thickened. Cream margarine until light and fluffy. Create sweetener by combining sorbitol and sugar replacement in a bowl, stirring to mix. Gradually add sweetener to creamed margarine, beating constantly. Continue beating until light and fluffy. Add vanilla and eggs, one at a time, beating well after each addition. Beat in cocoa mixture. Sift dry ingredients together. Add dry ingredients and remaining milk alternately to the creamed mixture. (Begin and end with dry ingredients.) Beat well after each addition. Continue beating until smooth. Pour batter into two 9-in. (23-cm) round layer pans. Pans should be greased and their bottoms lined with greased waxed paper. Bake at 350 °F (175 °C) for 25 to 30 minutes or until done. Cool in pans for 5 minutes. Turn out onto rack, remove paper, and cool completely.

Yield: 24 servings
Exchange, 1 serving: 1 starch/bread
Calories, 1 serving: 82
Carbohydrates, 1 serving: 16

Golden Butter Cake

½ c.	butter	125 mL
¾ c.	sorbitol	190 mL
½ t.	lemon flavoring	2 mL
dash	mace	dash
1½ c.	sifted cake flour	375 mL
1½ t.	baking powder	7 mL
½ t.	salt	2 mL
4	eggs, well beaten	4

Cream butter until light and fluffy. Gradually add sorbitol to creamed butter. Beat constantly until light and fluffy. Add lemon flavoring and mace. Sift dry ingredients together, and add to creamed mixture alternately with eggs, beating well after each addition. (Begin and end with dry ingredients.) Pour batter into greased and floured 8-in. (20-cm) tube pan or greased and floured 9×5×3 in. (23×13×7 cm) loaf pan. Bake at 350 °F (175 °C) for 50 minutes or until cake tests done. Cool in pan for 5 minutes. Turn out onto rack, and cool completely.

Yield: 16 servings
Exchange, 1 serving: ¾ starch/bread, ¾ fat
Calories, 1 serving: 81
Carbohydrates, 1 serving: 8

Pink 'n' Pretty Cake

8 oz.	sugar-free white cake mix	227 g
1 env.	unsweetened raspberry-drink mix	1 env.
2 c.	water	750 mL
1 T.	cornstarch	15 mL
4 env.	aspartame low-calorie sweetener	4 env.

Make cake as directed on package in an 8-in. (20-cm) round cake pan. Combine drink mix, water, and cornstarch in a small saucepan. Stir to mix. Cook over medium heat until thickened. Cool slightly; then stir in sweetener. Allow to set to jelly stage. Cut cake into three thin layers. Using half of the raspberry mixture, spread evenly over two of the layers. Chill thoroughly. Chill remaining raspberry mixture. When completely set, stack together the two raspberry-covered layers; then set the third layer on top, and frost top of cake with remaining raspberry mixture. Store in refrigerator.

Yield: 10 servings
Exchange, 1 serving: 1¼ starch/bread
Calories, 1 serving: 100
Carbohydrates, 1 serving: 18

Marble Cake

½ c.	solid vegetable shortening	125 mL
1½ c.	granulated sugar replacement	375 mL
2 t.	vanilla extract	10 mL
2 c.	sifted cake flour	500 mL
1 t.	salt	5 mL
2 t.	baking powder	10 mL
½ c.	skim milk	125 mL
4	egg whites, stiffly beaten	4
2 sq. (1 oz. each)	unsweetened chocolate, melted	2 sq. (30 g each)
3 T.	water	45 mL

Cream shortening. Gradually add 1¼ c. (310 mL) of the sugar replacement, beating until light and fluffy. Beat in vanilla. Sift the dry ingredients together. Add dry ingredients alternately with the milk to the creamed mixture. (Begin and end with the dry ingredients.) Fold in the stiffly beaten egg whites. Divide batter in half. Now add remaining sugar replacement to melted chocolate in a saucepan. Blend in water. Cook and stir over low heat until mixture becomes thick. Allow to cool and then blend into half of the batter. Alternate layers of light and chocolate in well greased, waxed-paper-lined 9×5×3 in. (23×13×7 cm) loaf pan. Cut through layers of batter to produce a marbling effect. Bake at 350 °F (175 °C) for 60 minutes or until done. Turn out onto rack, remove paper, and cool completely.

Yield: 16 servings
Exchange, 1 serving: 1 starch/bread, 1⅓ fat
Calories, 1 serving: 128
Carbohydrates, 1 serving: 16

Quick Peanut-Butter Cake

8 oz.	sugar-free white cake mix	227 g
⅔ c.	water	180 mL
1	egg white	1
⅓ c.	crunchy peanut butter	90 mL

Empty cake mix into a bowl. Add water, egg white, and peanut butter. Blend for 4 to 5 minutes or until creamy. Transfer to 8-in. (20-cm) greased cake pan. Bake at 350 °F (175 °C) for 20 to 25 minutes. Allow cake to cool, then remove from pan.

Yield: 10 servings
Exchange, 1 serving: 1 starch/bread, 1½ fat
Calories, 1 serving: 125
Carbohydrates, 1 serving: 18

Quick Applesauce Cake

8 oz.	sugar-free white cake mix	227 g
1 c.	unsweetened applesauce	250 mL
1	egg white	1

Empty cake mix into a bowl. Add applesauce and egg white. Blend for 5 to 6 minutes or until creamy. Transfer to 8-in. (20-cm) greased cake pan. Bake at 350 °F (175 °C) for 20 to 25 minutes. Allow cake to cool; then remove from pan.

Yield: 10 servings
Exchange, 1 serving: 1 starch/bread, 1 fat
Calories, 1 serving: 110
Carbohydrates, 1 serving: 20

Lemon Cream Cake

8 oz.	sugar-free white cake mix	227 g
⅔ c.	water	180 mL
1	egg	1
1 T.	grated lemon zest	15 mL
1 t.	lemon flavoring	5 mL
1 env.	nondairy whipped-topping mix	1 env.
½ c.	water	125 mL
2 t.	cornstarch	10 mL
1 t.	orange flavoring	5 mL
⅛ t.	almond extract	½ mL

Empty cake mix into a bowl. Add ⅔-c. (180-mL) water, egg, lemon zest, and lemon flavoring. Beat for 4 to 5 minutes or until creamy. Transfer to 8-in. (20-cm) greased cake pan. Bake at 350 °F (175 °C) fo 20 to 25 minutes. Allow cake to cool; then remove from pan. In a chilled bowl and using a chilled beater, beat whipped-topping mix and ½-c. (125-mL) water until soft peaks form. Gradually beat in cornstarch and flavorings. Beat to stiff peaks. Frost cake.

Yield: 10 servings
Exchange, 1 serving: 1⅓ starch/bread, 1 fat
Calories, 1 serving: 132
Carbohydrates, 1 serving: 22

Cake de Menthe

8 oz.	sugar-free white cake mix	227 g
½ c.	water	125 mL
3 T.	crème de menthe	45 mL
1	egg white	1

Empty cake mix into a bowl. Add water, crème de menthe, and egg white. Beat for 4 to 5 minutes or until creamy. Transfer to 8-in. (20-cm) greased cake pan. Bake 350 °F (175 °C) for 20 to 25 minutes. Allow cake to cool; then remove from pan.

Yield: 10 servings
Exchange, 1 serving: 1 starch/bread, 1 fat
Calories, 1 serving: 104
Carbohydrates, 1 serving: 19

Cake de Cacao

8 oz.	sugar-free white cake mix	227 g
½ c.	water	125 mL
2 T.	crème de cacao	30 mL
1 T.	vanilla extract	15 mL
1 t.	cocoa powder	5 mL
1	egg white	1

Empty cake mix into a bowl. Add water, crème de cacao, vanilla, cocoa, and egg white. Beat for 4 to 5 minutes or until creamy. Transfer to 8-in. (20-cm) greased cake pan. Bake at 350 °F (175 °C) for 20 to 25 minutes. Allow cake to cool; then remove from pan.

Yield: 10 servings
Exchange, 1 serving: 1 starch/bread, 1 fat
Calories, 1 serving: 102
Carbohydrates, 1 serving: 18

Coconut Cream Cake

8 oz.	sugar-free white cake mix	227 g
⅔ c.	water	180 mL
1	egg white	1
½ c.	unsweetened shredded coconut, toasted	125 mL
2 c.	prepared nondairy whipped topping	500 mL

Empty cake mix into a bowl. Add water and egg white. Beat for 4 to 5 minutes or until smooth. Fold in ⅓ c. (90 mL) of the toasted coconut. Transfer to 8-in. (20-cm) greased cake pan, Bake at 350 °F (175 °C) for 20 to 25 minutes. Allow cake to cool, and then remove from pan. Cut cake in half horizontally. Place one-half of cake on serving plate. Frost top with some of the nondairy whipped topping. Arrange second layer on top of first layer. Completely frost top and sides of cake. Then sprinkle with remaining toasted coconut. Refrigerate at least 30 minutes before serving.

Yield: 10 servings
Exchange, 1 serving: 1 starch/bread, 1 fat
Calories, 1 serving: 121
Carbohydrates, 1 serving: 21

Mocha Almond Cake

8 oz.	sugar-free chocolate cake mix	227 g
⅔ c.	strong coffee	180 mL
1	egg	1
2 t.	almond extract	10 mL
¼ c.	toasted slivered almonds	60 mL

Empty cake mix into a bowl. Add coffee, egg, and almond extract. Beat for 4 to 5 minutes or until creamy. Fold in toasted almonds. Transfer to 8-in. (20-cm) greased cake pan. Bake at 350 °F (175 °C) for 20 to 25 minutes. Allow cake to cool; then remove from pan.

Yield: 10 servings
Exchange, 1 serving: 1 starch/bread, 1 fat
Calories, 1 serving: 117
Carbohydrates, 1 serving: 18

Chocolate Coconut Pecan Cake

8 oz.	sugar-free chocolate cake mix	227 g
⅔ c.	water	180 mL
1	egg white	1
¼ c.	unsweetened grated coconut	60 mL
2 T.	chopped pecans	30 mL

Empty cake mix into a bowl. Add water and egg white. Beat for 4 to 5 minutes or until creamy. Fold in coconut and pecans. Transfer to 8-in. (20-cm) greased cake pan. Bake at 350 °F (175 °C) for 20 to 25 minutes. Allow cake to cool; then remove from pan.

Yield: 10 servings
Exchange, 1 serving: 1 starch/bread, 1 fat
Calories, 1 serving: 102
Carbohydrates, 1 serving: 18

Dark-Cherry Chocolate Cake

8 oz.	sugar-free chocolate cake mix	227 g
⅔ c.	water	180 mL
1	egg white	1
½ t.	almond extract	2 mL
¼ c.	chopped dark cherries	60 mL

Empty cake mix into a bowl. Add water, egg white, and almond extract.

Beat for 4 to 5 minutes or until creamy. Fold in chopped cherries. Transfer to 8-in. (20-cm) greased cake pan. Bake at 350 °F (175 °C) for 20 to 25 minutes. Allow cake to cool; then remove from pan.

Yield: 10 servings
Exchange, 1 serving: 1 starch/bread, 1 fat
Calories, 1 serving: 104
Carbohydrates, 1 serving: 18

Pumpkin Carrot Cake

8 oz.	sugar-free white cake mix	227 g
⅓ c.	water	90 mL
⅓ c.	carrot purée*	90 mL
1	egg	1
2 t.	pumpkin-pie spice	10 mL

*Baby-food carrot purée can be used.

Empty cake mix into a bowl. Add remaining ingredients. Beat for 4 to 5 minutes or until creamy. Transfer to 8-in. (20-cm) greased cake pan. Bake at 350 °F (175 °C) for 20 to 25 minutes. Allow cake to cool; then remove from pan.

Yield: 10 servings
Exchange, 1 serving: 1 starch/bread, 1 fat
Calories, 1 serving: 102
Carbohydrates, 1 serving: 18

Chocolate Brandy Cake

8 oz.	sugar-free chocolate cake mix	227 g
⅔ c.	buttermilk	180 mL
1	egg white	1
1 t.	brandy flavoring	2 mL

Empty cake mix into a bowl. Add buttermilk, egg white, and brandy flavoring. Beat for 4 to 5 minutes or until creamy. Transfer to 8-in. (20-cm) greased cake pan. Bake at 350 °F (175 °C) for 20 to 25 minutes. Allow cake to cool; then remove from pan.

Yield: 10 servings
Exchange, 1 serving: 1 starch/bread, 1 fat
Calories, 1 serving: 106
Carbohydrates, 1 serving: 18

Chocolate Sour-Cream Raisin Cake

8 oz.	sugar-free chocolate cake mix	227 g
¼ c.	granulated brown-sugar replacement	60 mL
3 T.	granulated sugar replacement	45 mL
1 T.	cornstarch	15 mL
½ c.	low-calorie sour cream	125 mL
1	egg yolk	1
¼ c.	raisins	60 mL
1 t.	vanilla extract	5 mL

Bake cake from mix as directed on package. Allow cake to cool completely. In a small saucepan, mix sugar replacements and cornstarch. Blend in sour cream and egg yolk. Cool and stir over medium heat until mixture thickens and boils. Boil and stir for 1 minute longer. Remove from heat. Stir in raisins and vanilla. Cool completely. Frost cake.

Yield: 10 servings
Exchange, 1 serving: 1 starch/bread, 1 fat
Calories, 1 serving: 134
Carbohydrates, 1 serving: 19

Easy Chocolate Crunch Cake

8 oz.	chocolate cake mix	227 g
⅔ c.	water	180 mL
1	egg white	1
⅓ c.	wheat and barley cereal	90 mL

Empty cake mix into a bowl. Add water and egg white. Beat for 4 to 5 minutes or until creamy. Fold in cereal. Transfer to 8-in. (20-cm) greased cake pan. Bake at 350 °F (175 °C) for 20 to 25 minutes. Allow cake to cool; then remove from pan.

Yield: 10 servings
Exchange, 1 serving: 1 starch/bread, 1 fat
Calories, 1 serving: 103
Carbohydrates, 1 serving: 17

Pies

Blueberry Pie

	unbaked double crust	
4 c.	frozen unsweetened blueberries, thawed	1000 mL
½ c.	granulated sugar replacement	125 mL
⅓ c.	all-purpose flour	90 mL
1 t.	grated lemon peel	5 mL
dash	salt	dash
1 T.	low-calorie margarine, melted	15 mL

Combine blueberries, sugar replacement, flour, lemon peel, salt, and melted margarine in a large bowl. Toss to mix. Transfer to 9-in. (23-cm) pastry-lined pie pan. Adjust top crust, flute or pinch edges, and cut slits in top to allow steam to escape. Bake at 425 °F (220 °C) for 40 to 50 minutes or until lightly browned.

Yield: 8 servings
Exchange, 1 serving (without crust): 1 fruit
Calories, 1 serving (without crust): 68
Carbohydrates, 1 serving (without crust): 14

Gooseberry Pie

	unbaked double crust	
3 c.	gooseberries	750 mL
¾ c.	granulated fructose	190 mL
3½ T.	quick-cooking tapioca	52 mL
1 T.	low-calorie margarine	15 mL

Slightly crush the gooseberries. Stir in fructose and tapioca. Transfer to 9-in. (23-cm) pastry-lined pie pan. Dot with margarine. Adjust top crust, flute or pinch edges, and cut slits in top to allow steam to escape. Bake at 425 °F (220 °C) for 40 to 45 minutes or until lightly browned.

Yield: 8 servings
Exchange, 1 serving (without crust): 2 fruits
Calories, 1 serving (without crust): 122
Carbohydrates, 1 serving (without crust): 28

Wild-Blueberry Pie

9 in.	baked pie shell	23 cm
5 T.	granulated fructose	75 mL
3 T.	cornstarch	45 mL
dash	salt	dash
¼ c.	water	60 mL
1 qt.	wild blueberries*	1 L
1 T.	low-calorie margarine	15 mL

*Fresh cultivated blueberries can be substituted for wild blueberries.

Combine fructose, cornstarch, and salt in heavy nonstick saucepan. Add water and 1½ c. (375 mL) of the blueberries. Cook over medium heat until mixture thickens. Remove from heat and stir in margarine. Pour remaining 2½ c. (625 mL) of the blueberries into bottom of baked shell. Top with blueberry glaze. Chill thoroughly.

Yield: 8 servings
Exchange, 1 serving (without crust): 1 fruit, ⅓ fat
Calories, 1 serving (without crust): 75
Carbohydrates, 1 serving (without crust): 16

Summer Mulberry Pie

	unbaked double crust	
5 T.	granulated fructose	75 mL
¼ c.	all-purpose flour	60 mL
2 T.	cornstarch	30 mL
dash	salt	dash
1 qt.	mulberries, cleaned	1 L
2 T.	low-calorie margarine	30 mL

Combine fructose, flour, cornstarch, and salt in a bowl. Toss to mix. Sprinkle half of mixture into bottom of 9-in. (23-cm) pastry-lined pie pan. Fill with mulberries. Sprinkle remaining mixture over top. Dot with margarine. Adjust top crust, flute or pinch edges, and cut slits in top to allow steam to escape. Bake at 425 °F (220 °C) for 40 to 50 minutes or until lightly browned.

Yield: 8 servings
Exchange, 1 serving (without crust): 1 fruit, ½ fat
Calories, 1 serving (without crust): 91
Carbohydrates, 1 serving (without crust): 17

Fresh-Elderberry Pie

	unbaked double crust	
4 c.	elderberries, cleaned	1000 mL
1 T.	cider vinegar	15 mL
½ c.	granulated sugar replacement	125 mL
⅓ c.	all-purpose flour	90 mL
2 t.	cornstarch	10 mL
dash	salt	dash

Place elderberries into bottom of 9-in. (23-cm) pastry-lined pie pan. Sprinkle with vinegar. Combine sugar replacement, flour, cornstarch, and salt in medium-size bowl. Stir to blend. Sprinkle mixture over berries. Adjust top crust, flute or pinch edges, and cut slits in top to allow steam to escape. Bake at 400 °F (200 °C) for 35 to 45 minutes or until lightly browned.

Yield: 8 servings
Exchange, 1 serving (without crust): 1 fruit
Calories, 1 serving (without crust): 69
Carbohydrates, 1 serving (without crust): 15

Purple-Plum Pie

9 in.	unbaked pie shell	23 cm
1 qt.	sliced purple plums	1 L
⅓ c.	granulated sugar replacement	90 mL
¼ c.	all-purpose flour	60 mL
2 t.	cider vinegar	10 mL

Combine plums, sugar replacement, flour, and cider vinegar in a large bowl. Toss to mix. Transfer to pie shell. Place pie in a baking bag, and fasten bag securely. Bake at 425 °F (220 °C) for 50 to 60 minutes. Remove bag from oven. Allow pie to cool inside the bag until lukewarm. Remove pie from bag to cooling rack.

Yield: 8 servings
Exchange, 1 serving (without crust): 1 fruit
Calories, 1 serving (without crust): 58
Carbohydrates, 1 serving (without crust): 15

Fresh-Raspberry Pie

	baked pie shell	
1 qt.	fresh raspberries	1 L
1 c.	cold water	250 mL
½ c.	granulated fructose	125 mL
3 T.	cornstarch	45 mL
1 t.	fresh lemon juice	5 mL

Wash and thoroughly drain raspberries. Combine 1 c. (250 mL) of the raspberries, water, fructose, and cornstarch in nonstick saucepan. Stir to blend. Cook and stir over medium heat until thickened. Remove from heat and add lemon juice. Cool to lukewarm. Pour the remaining 3 c. (750 mL) of drained raspberries into bottom of baked pie shell. Top with raspberry glaze. Chill until firm.

Yield: 8 servings
Exchange, 1 serving (without crust): 1 fruit
Calories, 1 serving (without crust): 68
Carbohydrates, 1 serving (without crust): 16

Cranberry Relish Pie

	unbaked double Cheddar-cheese crust	
2½ c.	ground cranberries	625 mL
1 c.	ground Golden Delicious apples (unpeeled)	250 mL
½ c.	ground orange pulp and peel	125 mL
¾ c.	granulated fructose	190 mL
3 T.	all-purpose flour	45 mL
¼ t. each	cinnamon and nutmeg	1 mL each
2 T.	low-calorie margarine	30 mL

Combine fruits, fructose, flour, cinnamon, and nutmeg in a bowl. Toss to mix. Transfer to 9-in. (23-cm) pastry-lined pie pan. Dot with margarine. Adjust top crust, flute or pinch edges, and cut slits in top to allow steam to escape. Bake at 425 °F (220 °C) for 40 to 50 minutes or until lightly browned.

Yield: 8 servings
Exchange, 1 serving (without crust): 2 fruits
Calories, 1 serving (without crust): 112
Carbohydrates, 1 serving (without crust): 25

White-Grape Pie

8 in.	baked pie shell	20 cm
3 c.	seedless white grapes	750 mL
2 c.	white-grape juice	500 mL
3 T.	cornstarch	45 mL
1 t.	clear vanilla flavoring	5 mL

Wash grapes. Place grapes in a strainer, and pour 1 qt. (1 L) of boiling water over them. Drain thoroughly. Combine white-grape juice and cornstarch in a saucepan. Cook and stir over medium heat until mixture is clear and thickened. Remove from heat and stir in vanilla flavoring. (A small drop of green food coloring can be added, if desired.) Allow to cool to lukewarm. Place well drained grapes into bottom of pie shell. Pour juice mixture over the top. Chill until firm.

Yield: 8 servings
Exchange, 1 serving (without crust): 2 fruits
Calories, 1 serving (without crust): 118
Carbohydrates, 1 serving (without crust): 29

Fresh-Strawberry Pie

8 in.	baked pie shell	20 cm
1½ qts.	fresh strawberries	1½ L
½ c.	cold water	125 mL
4 T.	xylitol	60 mL
3 T.	cornstarch	45 mL

Clean and thoroughly drain strawberries. Combine 2 c. (500 mL) of the strawberries and the water in nonstick saucepan. Mash slightly with the back of a spoon or potato masher. Add xylitol and cornstarch. Stir to blend. Cook and stir over medium heat until mixture is clear and thickened. Remove from heat and cool to lukewarm. Place remaining 1 qt. (1 L) of strawberries in bottom of baked pie shell. Pour strawberry glaze over the top. Chill until firm. (A few drops of red food coloring can be added to the glaze, if desired.)

Yield: 8 servings
Exchange, 1 serving (without crust): 1 fruit
Calories, 1 serving (without crust): 62
Carbohydrates, 1 serving (without crust): 14

Fresh-Tart-Cherry Pie

	unbaked double crust	
½ c.	granulated fructose	125 mL
⅓ c.	all-purpose flour	90 mL
¼ c.	granulated sugar replacement	60 mL
1 qt.	pitted tart cherries	1 L
2 or 3 drops	almond extract	2 or 3 drops
2 T.	low-calorie margarine	30 mL

Combine fructose, flour, and sugar replacement in a large bowl. Add cherries and almond extract. Toss to coat. Transfer cherry mixture to bottom of 9-in. (23-cm) pastry-lined pie pan. Dot with margarine. Adjust top crust, flute or pinch edges, and cut slits in top to allow steam to escape. Bake at 425 °F (220 °C) for 40 to 50 minutes or until lightly browned.

Yield: 8 servings
Exchange, 1 serving (without crust): 1 fruit, ⅓ bread
Calories, 1 serving (without crust): 106
Carbohydrates, 1 serving (without crust): 22

Fresh-Sweet-Cherry Pie

9 in.	baked pie shell	23 cm
1 qt.	pitted sweet cherries	1 L
½ c.	granulated sugar replacement	125 mL
3 T.	cornstarch	45 mL
dash	salt	dash
1 t.	lemon juice	5 mL

Place sweet cherries in medium-size bowl. With the back of a spoon, push to extract the juice. Drain juice into medium-size saucepan. Reserve cherries. Add sugar replacement, cornstarch, and salt to cherry juice in saucepan. Stir to blend. Cook and stir over medium heat until clear and thickened. Remove from heat, and stir in lemon juice. Cool to lukewarm. Fold cherries into cooled glaze. Chill to rethicken. Transfer to baked pie shell. Chill until firm.

Yield: 8 servings
Exchange, 1 serving (without crust): 1 fruit
Calories, 1 serving (without crust): 64
Carbohydrates, 1 serving (without crust): 15

Peach Pie

	unbaked double crust	
2 (1 lb.) cans	sliced peaches, in their own juice	2 (489 g) cans
2 T.	granulated fructose	30 mL
3 T.	cornstarch	45 mL
½ t.	nutmeg	2 mL
dash	salt	dash
⅛ t.	almond extract	½ mL

Drain juice from peaches into a saucepan by pushing down lightly on peaches in can. Transfer peaches from can to strainer, allowing any excess juice to run off. Add fructose, cornstarch, nutmeg, salt, and almond extract to juice in saucepan. Cook and stir over medium heat until clear and thickened. Arrange peaches in the bottom of a 9-in. (23-cm) pastry-lined pie pan. Pour juice mixture over peaches. Adjust top crust, and pinch or flute edges; then cut in vents to allow steam to escape. Bake at 400 °F (200 °C) for 40 to 45 minutes.

Yield: 8 servings
Exchange, 1 serving (without crust): 1 fruit
Calories, 1 serving (without crust): 66
Carbohydrates, 1 serving (without crust): 16

Applecot Pie

	unbaked double crust	
¼ c.	granulated sugar replacement	60 mL
1 T.	all-purpose flour	15 mL
½ t.	cinnamon	2 mL
dash	salt	dash
1 qt.	sliced apples (peeled)	1 L
1 c.	apricots, in their own juice	250 mL

Combine sugar replacement, flour, cinnamon, and salt in a large bowl. Add apples and toss to coat. Drain apricots. Fold in apricots. Transfer to 8- or 9-in. (20- or 23-cm) pastry-lined pie pan. Adjust top crust, and flute or pinch edges. Then score top to allow steam to escape. Bake at 400 °F (200 °C) for 40 to 50 minutes or until top becomes lightly browned.

Yield: 8 servings
Exchange, 1 serving (without crust): 1⅓ fruits
Calories, 1 serving (without crust): 76
Carbohydrates, 1 serving (without crust): 19

Old-Fashioned Apple Pie

	unbaked double crust	
2½ lbs.	apples	1 kg
2 t.	lemon juice	10 mL
⅓ c.	granulated fructose	90 mL
1½ t.	apple-pie spice	7 mL
2 T.	all-purpose flour	30 mL

Peel and core apples; then slice them into a medium-size bowl. Sprinkle lemon juice over apple slices. Toss to coat. Sprinkle fructose and apple-pie spice over apple slices. Toss to coat. Cover and allow to set for 20 minutes. Sprinkle flour over apple slices and toss to coat. Transfer apple mixture to 9-in. (23-cm) pastry-lined pie pan. Adjust top crust, and flute or pinch edges. Then score top to allow steam to escape. Bake at 425 °F (220 °C) for 50 to 60 minutes or until top becomes lightly browned.

Yield: 8 servings
Exchange, 1 serving (without crust): 1½ fruits
Calories, 1 serving (without crust): 94
Carbohydrates, 1 serving (without crust): 22

Green-Apple Pie

	unbaked double crust	
7 c.	sliced green apples (unpeeled)	1750 mL
½ c.	granulated fructose	125 mL
2 T.	apple juice	30 mL
3 T.	cornstarch	45 mL
1	egg white	1
1 t.	water	5 mL

Combine apple slices, fructose, apple juice, and cornstarch in a bowl. Toss to mix. Transfer to 9-in. (23-cm) pastry-lined pie pan. Adjust top crust, and flute or pinch edges. Then score top to allow steam to escape. Combine egg white and water, and beat slightly. Brush top crust with egg-water mixture. Bake at 425 °F (220 °C) for 50 to 60 minutes or until top becomes lightly browned.

Yield: 8 servings
Exchange, 1 serving (without crust): 2 fruits
Calories, 1 serving (without crust): 110
Carbohydrates, 1 serving (without crust): 27

Apple 'n' Cheese Pie

	unbaked double crust	
6 c.	sliced apples (peeled)	1500 mL
1 T.	apple juice	15 mL
⅓ c.	granulated fructose	90 mL
2 T.	all-purpose flour	30 mL
¾ t.	apple-pie spice	4 mL
¼ lb.	grated sharp Cheddar cheese	120 g

Combine apples and apple juice in bowl, and toss to mix. Combine fructose, flour, and apple-pie spice in another bowl. Stir to mix. Sprinkle a third of the fructose mixture on bottom of 8-in. (20-cm) pastry-lined deep-dish pie pan. Transfer apple and juice to pie pan. Sprinkle with remaining fructose mixture. Top with grated cheese. Adjust top crust, and flute or pinch edges. Then score top to allow steam to escape. Bake at 400 °F (200 °C) for 50 to 60 minutes or until top becomes lightly browned.

Yield: 8 servings
Exchange, 1 serving (without crust): 1½ fruits, ⅓ whole milk
Calories, 1 serving (without crust): 162
Carbohydrates, 1 serving (without crust): 27

Easy Apple Pie

1 recipe	Graham-Cracker Crust, unbaked	1 recipe
1½ lbs.	sliced Golden Delicious apples (peeled)	750 g
2 T.	granulated brown-sugar replacement	30 mL
1½ T.	all-purpose flour	21 mL
½ t.	cinnamon	2 mL

Combine apples, brown-sugar replacement, flour, and cinnamon in a bowl. Toss to coat apples. Press three-fourths of the Graham-Cracker Crust (page 133) into the bottom of an 8-in. (20-cm) tart pan with removable bottom. Transfer apple mixture over crust mixture in tart pan. Then sprinkle remaining crust mixture over top. Bake at 350 °F (175 °C) for 20 to 25 minutes or until top becomes lightly browned. Cool before serving.

Yield: 8 servings
Exchange, 1 serving (without crust): 1 fruit
Calories, 1 serving (without crust): 70
Carbohydrates, 1 serving (without crust): 18

Raspberry Apple Pie

	unbaked double crust	
3 c.	fresh raspberries	750 mL
1 c.	sliced Golden Delicious apples (peeled)	250 mL
3 T.	quick-cooking tapioca	45 mL
¾ c.	granulated sugar replacement	190 mL
½ t.	cinnamon	2 mL
1½ T.	low-calorie margarine	21 mL

Clean and drain raspberries. Combine raspberries, apples, tapioca, sugar replacement, and cinnamon in a large bowl. Toss to mix. Transfer to 9-in. (23-cm) pastry-lined pie pan. Dot with margarine. Adjust top crust, and flute or pinch edges. Then score top to allow steam to escape. Bake at 425 °F (220 °C) for 40 to 50 minutes or until top becomes lightly browned. (This also tastes good with a cheese crust.)

Yield: 8 servings
Exchange, 1 serving (without crust): 1 fruit
Calories, 1 serving (without crust): 58
Carbohydrates, 1 serving (without crust): 12

Summer's Best Fresh-Peach Pie

	unbaked double crust	
5 c.	sliced fresh peaches (peeled)	1250 mL
6 T.	granulated fructose	90 mL
2 T.	quick-cooking tapioca	30 mL
½ t.	lemon juice	2 mL
¼ t.	nutmeg	1 mL
⅛ t.	almond extract	½ mL
2 T.	low-calorie margarine	30 mL

Combine peaches, fructose, tapioca, lemon juice, nutmeg, and almond extract in a bowl. Toss to mix. Transfer to bottom of 9-in. (23-cm) pastry-lined pie pan. Dot with margarine. Adjust top crust, and pinch or flute edges; then cut in vents to allow steam to escape. Bake at 425 °F (220 °C) for 40 to 50 minutes.

Yield: 8 servings
Exchange, 1 serving (without crust): 1 fruit
Calories, 1 serving (without crust): 71
Carbohydrates, 1 serving (without crust): 14

Green-Grape and Apple Pie

	unbaked double crust	
2 c.	seedless green grapes	500 mL
3 large	Golden Delicious apples	3 large
1 large	Red Delicious apple	1 large
½ c.	granulated sugar replacement	125 mL
3 T.	quick-cooking tapioca	45 mL
½ t.	cardamom	2 mL
1 t.	vanilla extract	5 mL
dash	salt	dash
2 T.	low-calorie margarine	30 mL

Wash and sort grapes. Peel, core, and slice apples. Combine fruit, sugar replacement, tapioca, cardamom, vanilla, and salt in a large bowl. Toss to mix. Transfer to 9-in (23-cm) pastry-lined pie pan. Dot with margarine. Adjust top crust, and pinch or flute edges; then cut in vents to allow steam to escape. Bake at 425 °F (220 °C) for 50 to 60 minutes.

Yield: 8 servings
Exchange, 1 serving (without crust): 1 fruit, ½ fat
Calories, 1 serving (without crust): 75
Carbohydrates, 1 serving (without crust): 15

Nectarine Pie

	unbaked double crust	
5 c.	sliced nectarines (peeled)	1250 mL
1 t.	lemon juice	5 mL
½ c.	granulated fructose	125 mL
⅓ c.	all-purpose flour	90 mL
¼ t.	nutmeg	1 mL
1 T.	low-calorie margarine	15 mL

Combine nectarines, lemon juice, fructose, flour, and nutmeg in a large bowl. Toss to mix. Transfer to 9-in. (23-cm) pastry-lined pie pan. Dot with margarine. Adjust top crust, and pinch or flute edges; then cut in vents to allow steam to escape. Bake at 425 °F (220 °C) for 40 to 50 minutes.

Yield: 8 servings
Exchange, 1 serving (without crust): 1⅔ fruits
Calories, 1 serving (without crust): 104
Carbohydrates, 1 serving (without crust): 24

Fresh-Pineapple Pie

	unbaked double crust	
3½ c.	fresh pineapple chunks	875 mL
2	eggs, slightly beaten	2
¾ c.	granulated sugar replacement	190 mL
2½ T.	all-purpose flour	37 mL
1 T.	grated lemon zest	15 mL
1 t.	lemon juice	5 mL
dash	salt	dash

Put pineapple chunks in bottom of 9-in. (23-cm) pastry-lined pie pan. Combine eggs, sugar replacement, flour, lemon zest, lemon juice, and salt in bowl. Beat to blend. Pour over pineapple chunks. Adjust top crust, and pinch or flute edges; then cut in vents to allow steam to escape. Bake at 425 °F (220 °C) for 40 to 50 minutes.

Yield: 8 servings
Exchange, 1 serving (without crust): 1 fruit
Calories, 1 serving (without crust): 63
Carbohydrates, 1 serving (without crust): 10

Strawberry and Rhubarb Pie

	unbaked double crust	
⅔ c.	sorbitol	180 mL
⅓ c.	all-purpose flour	90 mL
½ t.	grated fresh orange zest	2 mL
2 c.	fresh strawberries	500 mL
2 c.	cubed fresh rhubarb	500 mL
2 T.	low-calorie margarine	30 mL

Combine sorbitol, flour, and orange zest in a bowl. Stir to mix. Place half of the strawberries and half of the rhubarb in the bottom of a 9-in. (23-cm) pastry-lined pie pan. Sprinkle with half of the sorbitol-flour mixture. Arrange the remaining fruit in the pie pan. Sprinkle with remaining sorbitol-flour mixture. Dot with margarine. Adjust top crust, and pinch or flute edges, then cut in vents to allow steam to escape. Bake at 425 °F (220 °C) for 40 to 50 minutes.

Yield: 8 servings
Exchange, 1 serving (without crust): ½ fruit
Calories, 1 serving (without crust): 25
Carbohydrates, 1 serving (without crust): 7

Fresh-Rhubarb Pie

	unbaked double crust	
1 qt.	strawberry rhubarb	1 L
¾ c.	granulated fructose	190 mL
⅓ c.	all-purpose flour	90 mL
dash	salt	dash
2 T.	low-calorie margarine	30 mL

Clean rhubarb and then cut it into small chunks. Combine rhubarb, fructose, flour, and salt in a bowl. Toss to mix. Transfer to 9-in. (23-cm) pastry-lined pie pan. Dot with margarine. Adjust top crust, and pinch or flute edges; then cut in vents to allow steam to escape. Bake at 425 °F (220 °C) for 40 to 50 minutes.

Yield: 8 servings
Exchange, 1 serving (without crust): 1 fruit
Calories, 1 serving (without crust): 61
Carbohydrates, 1 serving (without crust): 14

Dried-Fruit Pie

	unbaked double crust	
½ c.	dried apricots	125 mL
½ c.	dried prunes	125 mL
⅓ c.	raisins	90 mL
¼ c.	orange juice	60 mL
⅛ t.	mace	½ mL

Pour boiling water over apricots and prunes, and allow to sit for 3 minutes. Drain and cover with a bath of cold water. Allow to soften for 3 hours. Then drain the liquid into a saucepan. Cut fruit into quarters, and put in saucepan with liquid. Cook and stir until fruit is completely softened and liquid is reduced to about ⅓ c. (90 mL). Remove from heat, and stir in raisins, orange juice, and mace. Transfer to 8-or 9-in. (20- or 23-cm) pastry-lined pie pan. Adjust top crust, and pinch or flute edges; then cut in vents to allow steam to escape. Bake at 400 °F (200 °C) for 30 to 35 minutes.

Yield: 8 servings
Exchange, 1 serving (without crust): 1 fruit
Calories, 1 serving (without crust): 60
Carbohydrates, 1 serving (without crust): 15

Cream Pie

8 in.	baked pie shell	20 cm
⅓ c.	granulated sugar replacement	90 mL
3 T.	cornstarch	45 mL
dash	salt	dash
½ c.	cold skim milk	125 mL
1½ c.	scalded skim milk	375 mL
3	egg yolks, beaten	3
2 t.	vanilla extract	10 mL
1 recipe	meringue topping	1 recipe

Combine sugar replacement, cornstarch, and salt in the top of a double boiler. Stir in cold milk to dissolve cornstarch. Slowly add scalded milk. Place over hot water. Cook and stir until mixture thickens. Pour small amount of thickened mixture into beaten egg yolks, stirring to mix. Return to pan. Cook 4 to 5 minutes longer. Stir in vanilla. Remove from heat and allow to cool. Transfer to baked pie shell. Top with meringue, sealing edges. (There are three meringue-topping recipes in this book [on pages 144–145]; use any one.) Bake at 350 °F (175 °C) for 7 to 10 minutes or until peaks are browned.

Yield: 8 servings
Exchange, 1 serving (without crust): 1 low-fat milk
Calories, 1 serving (without crust): 58
Carbohydrates, 1 serving (without crust): 6

Apricot Cream Pie

8 in.	baked pie shell	20 cm
¼ c.	granulated sugar replacement	60 mL
3 T.	cornstarch	45 mL
dash	salt	dash
½ c.	cold skim milk	125 mL
1½ c.	scalded skim milk	375 mL
3	egg yolks, beaten	3
1 c.	apricot purée	250 mL
½ t.	vanilla extract	2 mL
2 c.	prepared nondairy whipped topping	500 mL

Combine sugar replacement, cornstarch, and salt in the top of a double boiler. Stir in cold milk to dissolve cornstarch. Slowly add scalded milk. Place over hot water. Cook and stir until mixture thickens. Pour small amount of thickened mixture into beaten egg yolks, stirring to mix. Return to pan. Cook 4 to 5 minutes longer. Stir in apricot purée and vanilla. Cook for 2 minutes. Remove from heat and allow to cool. Transfer to baked pie shell. Cool thoroughly. Top with nondairy whipped topping.

Yield: 8 servings
Exchange, 1 serving (without crust): ¾ fruit, ½ low-fat milk
Calories, 1 serving (without crust): 103
Carbohydrates, 1 serving (without): 18

Fresh-Peach Cream Pie

8 in.	baked pie shell	20 cm
4	fresh peaches	4
2 t.	lemon juice	10 mL
¼ c.	granulated fructose	60 mL
3 T.	cornstarch	45 mL
dash	salt	dash
½ c.	cold skim milk	125 mL
1½ c.	scalded skim milk	375 mL
3	egg yolks, beaten	3
1 t.	almond extract	5 mL

Pour boiling water over peaches. Peel, remove the pits, and cut into thin slices. Place sliced peaches into a bowl of ice water; then add lemon juice and stir. Combine fructose, cornstarch, and salt in the top of a double boiler. Stir in cold milk to dissolve cornstarch. Slowly add scalded milk. Place over hot water. Cook and stir until mixture thickens. Pour small amount of thickened mixture into beaten egg yolks, stirring to mix. Return to pan. Cook 4 to 5 minutes longer. Stir in almond extract. Remove from heat and allow to cool. Transfer to baked pie shell. Chill until top becomes firm. Thoroughly drain peach slices and then pat them dry. Arrange peach slices on top of pie.

Yield: 8 servings
Exchange, 1 serving (without crust): ⅓ fruit, ½ low-fat milk
Calories, 1 serving (without crust): 78
Carbohydrates, 1 serving (without crust): 11

Pineapple Cream Pie

9 in.	baked pie shell	23 cm
1½ c.	crushed pineapple, in its own juice	375 mL
2 t.	cornstarch	10 mL
⅓ c.	granulated sugar replacement	90 mL
3 T.	cornstarch	45 mL
dash	salt	dash
½ c.	cold skim milk	125 mL
1½ c.	scalded skim milk	375 mL
3	egg yolks, beaten	3
1 t.	vanilla extract	5 mL
2 T.	grated semi-sweet chocolate	30 mL

Combine pineapple with juice and the 2-t. (10-mL) cornstarch in a saucepan. Stir to blend. Cook and stir over medium heat until mixture thickens. Set aside. Combine sugar replacement, the 3-T. (45-mL) cornstarch, and salt in the top of a double boiler. Stir in cold milk to dissolve cornstarch. Slowly add scalded milk. Place over hot water. Cook and stir until mixture thickens. Pour small amount of thickened mixture into beaten egg yolks, stirring to mix. Return to pan. Cook 4 to 5 minutes longer. Stir in vanilla. Remove from heat and allow to slightly cool. Pour just enough of the cream filling into pie shell to cover bottom. Spread pineapple filling on top. Allow to cool. Top with remaining cream filling. Then garnish with grated semi-sweet chocolate.

Yield: 8 servings
Exchange, 1 serving (without crust): ⅓ fruit, ½ low-fat milk
Calories, 1 serving (without crust): 76
Carbohydrates, 1 serving (without crust): 6

Banana Cream Pie

8 in.	baked pie shell	20 cm
⅓ c.	granulated fructose	90 mL
3 T.	cornstarch	45 mL
dash	salt	dash
½ c.	cold skim milk	125 mL
1½ c.	scalded skim milk	375 mL
3	egg yolks, beaten	3
2 t.	vanilla extract	10 mL

| 3 | sliced ripe bananas | 3 |
| 1 recipe | meringue topping | 1 recipe |

Combine fructose, cornstarch, and salt in the top of a double boiler. Stir in cold milk to dissolve cornstarch. Slowly add scalded milk. Place over hot water. Cook and stir until mixture thickens. Pour small amount of thickened mixture into beaten egg yolks, stirring to mix. Return to pan. Cook 4 to 5 minutes longer. Stir in vanilla. Remove from heat and allow to cool completely. Alternate layers of sliced bananas and cream filling in pie shell, ending with bananas. Top with meringue, sealing edges. (There are three meringue-topping recipes in this book [pages 144–145]; you can use any one of them.) Bake at 350 °F (175 °C) for 5 to 7 minutes or until peaks become slightly browned.

Yield: 8 servings
Exchange, 1 serving (without crust): ¾ fruit, ½ low-fat milk
Calories, 1 serving (without crust): 95
Carbohydrates, 1 serving (without crust): 16

Raspberry Cream Pie

9 in.	baked pie shell	23 cm
1½ c.	skim milk	375 mL
¼ c.	granulated sugar replacement	60 mL
¼ t.	salt	1 mL
3 T.	all-purpose flour	45 mL
1	egg yolk, beaten	1
1 T.	low-calorie margarine	15 mL
½ t.	vanilla extract	2 mL
1 c.	fresh raspberries	250 mL
2 c.	prepared nondairy whipped topping	500 mL

Combine skim milk, sugar replacement, salt, and flour in a heavy saucepan. Cook and stir until mixture thickens. Stir small amount of mixture into beaten egg yolk; then return to saucepan. Cook and stir 1 or 2 minutes longer. Stir in margarine and vanilla. Remove from heat and allow to cool. Fold in fresh raspberries. Transfer to baked pie shell. Top with nondairy whipped topping. Chill.

Yield: 8 servings
Exchange, 1 serving (without crust): ¾ fruit
Calories, 1 serving (without crust): 47
Carbohydrates, 1 serving (without crust): 11

Strawberry Cream Pie

8 in.	baked pie shell	20 cm
2 c.	frozen unsweetened strawberries, thawed	500 mL
1½ c.	skim milk	375 mL
⅓ c.	granulated fructose	90 mL
4 T.	all-purpose flour	60 mL
2	egg yolks, beaten	2
1 t.	low-calorie margarine	5 mL
2 t.	unsweetened strawberry-drink mix	10 mL
2 c.	prepared nondairy whipped topping	500 mL

Combine thawed strawberries, skim milk, fructose, and flour in a heavy saucepan. Cook and stir until mixture thickens. Pour small amount of mixture into beaten egg yolks; then return to saucepan. Cook and stir 1 or 2 minutes longer. Stir in margarine and unsweetened strawberry-drink mix. Remove from heat and allow to cool. Transfer to baked pie shell. Top with nondairy whipped topping. Chill.

Yield: 8 servings
Exchange, 1 serving (without crust): ¾ fruit, ½ fat
Calories, 1 serving (without crust): 96
Carbohydrates, 1 serving (without crust): 10

Blackberry Cream Pie

8 in.	baked pie shell	20 cm
1½ c.	evaporated skim milk	375 mL
½ c.	granulated sugar replacement	125 mL
2 T.	cornstarch	30 mL
1 t.	lemon juice	5 mL
1½ c.	fresh blackberries	375 mL

Combine evaporated milk, sugar replacement, cornstarch, and lemon juice in the top of a double boiler. Stir to dissolve cornstarch. Place over simmering water; then cook and stir until mixture thickens. Allow to cool slightly; then fold in blackberries. Transfer to baked pie shell. Allow to cool.

Yield: 8 servings
Exchange, 1 serving (without crust): ¾ fruit
Calories, 1 serving (without crust): 45
Carbohydrates, 1 serving (without crust): 9

Raisin Sour-Cream Pie

8 in.	baked pie shell	20 cm
½ c.	all-purpose flour	125 mL
¾ c.	granulated sugar replacement	190 mL
½ c.	cold skim milk	125 mL
½ c.	buttermilk	125 mL
1 c.	dairy, or regular, sour cream	250 mL
½ c.	chopped raisins	125 mL
1 t.	lemon juice	5 mL
3	egg yolks, beaten	3
	nutmeg	

Mix flour, sugar replacement, skim milk, buttermilk, sour cream, raisins, and lemon juice in the top of a double boiler. Stir to blend thoroughly. Place over hot water; then cook and stir until mixture thickens. Pour small amount of mixture into beaten egg yolks; then return to boiler. Cook and stir 3 minutes longer. Remove from heat and allow to cool. Transfer to baked pie shell. Sprinkle with nutmeg. Allow to cool.

Yield: 8 servings
Exchange, 1 serving (without crust): 1 fruit, ⅓ starch/bread, 1 fat
Calories, 1 serving (without crust): 148
Carbohydrates, 1 serving (without crust): 14

Date Cream Pie

8 in.	unbaked pie shell	20 cm
1	egg	1
¼ c.	granulated fructose	60 mL
½ t.	salt	2 mL
1 c.	evaporated skim milk	250 mL
2 T.	lemon juice	30 mL
¾ c.	chopped dates	190 mL

Combine egg, fructose, salt, evaporated milk, lemon juice, and dates in a bowl. Stir to completely mix. Pour into unbaked pie shell. Bake at 425 °F (220 °C) for 10 minutes; then reduce heat to 300 °F (150 °C) and bake 15 to 20 minutes longer or until filling becomes firm.

Yield: 8 servings
Exchange, 1 serving (without crust): 1½ fruits
Calories, 1 serving (without crust): 99
Carbohydrates, 1 serving (without crust): 21

Sour-Cream Pie

8 in.	baked pie shell	20 cm
½ c.	all-purpose flour	125 mL
¾ c.	granulated sugar replacement	190 mL
½ t.	salt	2 mL
1 c.	cold skim milk	250 mL
1 c.	dairy, or regular, sour cream	250 mL
1 t.	lemon juice	5 mL
3	egg yolks, beaten	3

Mix flour, sugar replacement, salt, and skim milk in the top of a double boiler. Stir to blend thoroughly. Stir in sour cream and lemon juice. Place over hot water; then cook and stir until mixture thickens. Pour small amount of mixture into beaten egg yolks; then return to top of double boiler. Cook and stir 3 minutes longer. Remove from heat and allow to cool. Transfer to baked pie shell. Allow to cool.

Yield: 8 servings
Exchange, 1 serving (without crust): ¾ low-fat milk, 1 fat
Calories, 1 serving (without crust): 126
Carbohydrates, 1 serving (without crust): 7

Buttermilk Cream Pie

9 in.	unbaked pie shell	23 cm
2 T.	all-purpose flour	30 mL
1 T.	low-calorie margarine	15 mL
2	egg yolks	2
2 T.	granulated fructose	30 mL
1 c.	buttermilk	250 mL
1 t.	lemon juice	5 mL

Combine flour and margarine in a bowl. With a fork, blend together. Beat egg yolks and fructose together. Add flour mixture, and beat until well blended. Beat in buttermilk and lemon juice. Transfer to unbaked pie shell. Bake at 425 °F (220 °C) for 10 minutes. Reduce heat to 350 °F (175 °C) and bake 20 to 25 minutes longer or until filling becomes firm. Allow to cool.

Yield: 8 servings
Exchange, 1 serving (without crust): ⅓ low-fat milk
Calories, 1 serving (without crust): 45
Carbohydrates, 1 serving (without crust): 4

Coffee Cream Pie

9 in.	baked pie shell	23 cm
¼ c.	all-purpose flour	60 mL
⅓ c.	granulated fructose	90 mL
dash	salt	dash
1 c.	strong coffee	250 mL
1 c.	skim milk	250 mL
2	egg yolks, beaten	2
1 T.	low-calorie margarine	15 mL
1 recipe	meringue topping	1 recipe

Mix flour, fructose, and salt together in a saucepan. Add coffee and skim milk, stirring to blend. Cook and stir over medium heat until mixture thickens. Pour small amount of mixture into beaten egg yolks; then return to saucepan. Cook and stir 2 minutes longer. Remove from heat. Stir in margarine. Cool slightly. Transfer to baked pie shell. Top with meringue, sealing edges. (There are three meringue-topping recipes in this book [on pages 144–145]; you can use any one.) Bake at 350 °F (175 °C) for 7 to 10 minutes or until peaks are browned. Cool.

Yield: 8 servings
Exchange, 1 serving (without crust): 1 starch/bread
Calories, 1 serving (without crust): 81
Carbohydrates, 1 serving (without crust): 12

Cherry Cream Pie

8 in.	baked pie shell	20 cm
1 env.	unflavored gelatin	1 env
¼ c.	cold water	60 mL
1-lb. can	tart cherries, with juice	489-g can
½ c.	granulated sugar replacement	125 mL
1 c.	prepared nondairy whipped topping	250 mL

Combine gelatin and cold water. Allow gelatin to soften for 5 minutes. Combine cherries with juice and sugar replacement in a saucepan. Heat slightly. Stir in gelatin. Heat until gelatin becomes completely dissolved. Remove from heat and allow to cool. Fold in nondairy whipped topping. Transfer to baked pie shell. Allow to cool.

Yield: 8 servings
Exchange, 1 serving (without crust): ½ fruit
Calories, 1 serving (without crust): 32
Carbohydrates, 1 serving (without crust): 7

Mocha Cream Pie

9 in.	baked pie shell	23 cm
¼ c.	instant coffee, powdered	60 mL
2 c.	skim milk	500 mL
¾ c.	granulated sugar replacement	190 mL
⅓ c.	all-purpose flour	90 mL
1 oz.	baking chocolate, melted	30 g
2	eggs	2
1	egg yolk	1
1 t.	vanilla extract	5 mL

Combine coffee powder and milk in a heavy saucepan. Place over low heat, and allow milk to scald. Strain using either a coffee filter or a very small strainer. Combine sugar replacement and flour in a saucepan. Slowly stir in coffee-flavored milk. Cook and stir until mixture thickens. Stir in chocolate. Beat eggs and egg yolk together. Add small amount of hot mixture to eggs; then return to saucepan. Cook and stir 2 minutes longer. Remove from heat and stir in vanilla. Cool slightly. Transfer to baked pie shell. Cool completely.

Yield: 8 servings
Exchange, 1 serving (without crust): ½ low-fat milk, 1 fat
Calories, 1 serving (without crust): 99
Carbohydrates, 1 serving (without crust): 6

Old-Fashioned Pumpkin Pie

9 in.	unbaked pie shell	23 cm
1¼ c.	canned pumpkin	310 mL
⅓ c.	granulated fructose	90 mL
1 c.	evaporated skim milk	250 mL
2	eggs	2
1 T.	cornstarch	15 mL
2 T.	cold water	30 mL
1 t.	cinnamon	5 mL
½ t.	nutmeg	2 mL

| ¼ t. | salt | 1 mL |
| ¼ t. | ginger | 1 mL |

Combine pumpkin, fructose, evaporated milk, and eggs in a large bowl. Beat to blend. Blend cornstarch in cold water. Beat into pumpkin mixture. Beat in cinnamon, nutmeg, salt, and ginger. Pour into unbaked pie shell. Bake at 400 °F (200 °C) for 45 to 50 minutes or until knife inserted in center comes out clean.

Yield: 8 servings
Exchange, 1 serving (without crust): 1¼ fruit
Calories, 1 serving (without crust): 80
Carbohydrates, 1 serving (without crust): 18

Pecan Pumpkin Pie

9 in.	unbaked pie shell	23 cm
1-lb. can	canned pumpkin	458-g can
2	eggs	2
½ c.	granulated sugar replacement	125 mL
½ t.	salt	2 mL
1 t.	cinnamon	5 mL
½ t.	ginger	2 mL
¼ t.	cloves	1 mL
1½ c.	half-and-half	375 mL
1 recipe	Pecan Topping	1 recipe
3 T.	dietetic maple syrup	45 mL

Combine pumpkin, eggs, sugar replacement, salt, cinnamon, ginger, cloves, and half-and-half in a large bowl. Beat to blend thoroughly. Pour into unbaked pie shell. Bake at 400 °F (200 °C) for 45 to 50 minutes or until knife inserted in center comes out clean. Sprinkle with Pecan Topping (page 140) and dietetic maple syrup.

Yield: 8 servings
Exchange, 1 serving (without crust): ¾ low-fat milk, 1⅔ fat
Calories, 1 serving (without crust): 167
Carbohydrates, 1 serving (without crust): 9

Pumpkin Meringue Pie

9 in.	unbaked pie shell	23 cm
1½ c.	canned pumpkin	375 mL
1½ c.	skim milk	375 mL
3	eggs	3
⅔ c.	granulated brown-sugar replacement	180 mL
1¼ t.	cinnamon	6 mL
½ t. each	salt, ginger, nutmeg	2 mL each
1 recipe	meringue topping	1 recipe

Combine pumpkin, skim milk, eggs, brown-sugar replacement, and spices in a large bowl. Beat to blend. Pour into unbaked pie shell. Bake at 400 °F (200 °C) for 45 to 50 minutes or until knife inserted in center comes out clean. Cool slightly. Spread meringue over pie, sealing edges. (There are three meringue-topping recipes in this book [on pages 144–145]; you can use any one.) Bake at 350 °F (175 °C) for 10 to 12 minutes or until the peaks begin to brown.

Yield: 8 servings
Exchange, 1 serving (without crust): ½ low-fat milk
Calories, 1 serving (without crust): 63
Carbohydrates, 1 serving (without crust): 7

Sweet-Potato Pie

9 in.	unbaked pie shell	23 cm
2 c.	sweet-potato purée	500 mL
2	eggs	2
½ c.	granulated sugar replacement	125 mL
2 T.	dietetic maple syrup	30 mL
1 t.	vanilla extract	5 mL
½ t. each	cinnamon, nutmeg, salt	2 mL each
1½ c.	skim milk	375 mL
1 recipe	meringue topping	1 recipe

Combine sweet-potato purée, eggs, sugar replacement, maple syrup, vanilla, spices, and skim milk in a large bowl. Beat to blend. Pour into unbaked pie shell. Bake at 400 °F (200 °C) for 45 to 50 minutes or until knife inserted in center comes out clean. Cool slightly. Spread meringue over pie, sealing edges. (You can use any one of the three meringue-topping recipes on pages 144–145.) Bake at 350 °F (175 °C) for 10 to 12 minutes or until the peaks begin to brown.

Yield: 8 servings
Exchange, 1 serving (without crust): 1 fruit
Calories, 1 serving (without crust): 55
Carbohydrates, 1 serving (without crust): 12

Fresh-Sweet-Potato Pie

8 in.	unbaked pie shell	20 cm
1 T.	low-calorie margarine	15 mL
¼ c.	granulated fructose	60 mL
1½ c.	grated fresh sweet potatoes	375 mL
1 t.	lemon juice	5 mL
2	eggs	2
1 c.	skim milk	250 mL
¼ t. each	nutmeg, cinnamon, salt	1 mL each
1 recipe	meringue topping	1 recipe

Melt margarine in a small skillet. Sprinkle fructose into the melted margarine and allow to brown slightly. Remove from heat. Combine grated sweet potatoes and lemon juice in a large bowl. Toss to blend. Add melted margarine-fructose mixture, eggs, skim milk, and spices. Beat to blend. Pour into unbaked pie shell. Bake at 400 °F (200 °C) for 45 to 50 minutes or until knife inserted in center comes out clean. Cool slightly. Spread meringue over pie, sealing edges. (You can use any one of the three meringue-topping recipes on pages 144–145.) Bake at 350 °F (175 °C) for 10 to 12 minutes or until the peaks begin to brown.

Yield: 8 servings
Exchange, 1 serving (without crust): 1 fruit
Calories, 1 serving (without crust): 69
Carbohydrates, 1 serving (without crust): 15

Sliced-Yam Pie ✓

	unbaked double crust	
1 lb.	yams	500 g
2 medium	apples	2 medium
1 t.	lemon juice	5 mL
½ c.	granulated brown-sugar replacement	125 mL
3 T.	granulated fructose	45 mL
½ t.	cinnamon	2 mL
½ t.	ginger	2 mL
dash	salt	dash
⅛ t.	cloves	½ mL
3 T.	low-calorie margarine	45 mL
½ c.	skim milk	125 mL

Boil yams until half-cooked; then cool with cold running water. Peel and slice. Peel, core, and slice apples. Combine yam and apple slices in a bowl. Sprinkle with lemon juice. Combine brown-sugar replacement, fructose, cinnamon, ginger, salt, and cloves in a bowl. Stir to mix. Layer a third of the yam-and-apple slices mixture in the bottom of a 8- or 9-in. (20- or 23-cm) pastry-lined pie pan. Sprinkle with a third of the sugar-replacement mixture; then dot with 1 T. (15 mL) of the margarine. Repeat these layers two more times. Pour skim milk over entire surface. Adjust top crust and seal edges securely. Bake at 425 °F (220 °C) for 35 to 45 minutes or until yams become soft.

Yield: 8 servings
Exchange, 1 serving (without crust): ½ starch/bread, ½ fruit
Calories, 1 serving (without crust): 73
Carbohydrates, 1 serving (without crust): 15

Slip Custard Pie

9 in.	baked pie shell	23 cm
4	eggs, slightly beaten	4
2½ c.	warm skim milk	625 mL
¼ c.	granulated fructose	60 mL
1 t.	vanilla extract	5 mL

dash	salt	dash
½ t.	nutmeg	2 mL

Combine eggs, skim milk, fructose, vanilla, and salt in a bowl. Beat to blend. Pour mixture into a 9-in. (23-cm) pie pan. Sprinkle with nutmeg. Place the filled pie pan into another pan containing water. (Water should reach halfway up sides of pie pan.) Bake at 350 °F (175 °C) for 30 to 35 minutes or until knife inserted in center comes out clean. Cool to room temperature. Carefully loosen around the edge of the custard with a sharp knife or thin spatula. Gently shake pie pan to further loosen custard. Then slip custard from pie pan into baked pie shell.

Yield: 8 servings
Exchange, 1 serving (without crust): ½ medium-fat meat, ½ skim milk
Calories, 1 serving (without crust): 89
Carbohydrates 1 serving (without crust): 8

Coconut Custard Pie

9 in.	unbaked pie shell	23 cm
4	eggs, slightly beaten	4
2 c.	warm skim milk	500 mL
½ c.	granulated sugar replacement	125 mL
1 t.	vanilla extract	5 mL
⅔ c.	flaked coconut	180 mL

Combine eggs, skim milk, sugar replacement, and vanilla in a bowl. Beat to blend. Sprinkle ⅓ c. (90 mL) of the coconut on the bottom of the unbaked pie shell. Pour custard mixture over coconut. Top with remaining coconut. Bake at 350 °F (175 °C) for 30 to 35 minutes or until knife inserted in center comes out clean. Cool to room temperature.

Yield: 8 servings
Exchange, 1 serving (without crust): ½ medium-fat meat, 1 fat
Calories, 1 serving (without crust): 82
Carbohydrates, 1 serving (without crust): 4

Vanilla Pie

9 in.	baked pie shell, chilled	23 cm
¾ c.	granulated sugar replacement	190 mL
5 T.	cornstarch	75 mL
1½ c.	boiling water	375 mL
3	egg whites	3
dash	salt	dash
1 T.	vanilla extract	15 mL
1 c.	prepared nondairy whipped topping	250 mL

Combine sugar replacement and cornstarch in a heavy saucepan. Slowly add boiling water, stirring constantly. Cook and stir until clear and thickened. Combine egg whites and salt in a large mixing bowl. Beat until stiff. Then beat in vanilla. Continue beating until whites are creamy. Slowly pour cornstarch mixture over egg whites, beating continually. Cool slightly. Transfer to baked pie shell. Cool completely. Top with whipped topping.

Yield: 8 servings
Exchange, 1 serving (without crust): ½ starch/bread
Calories, 1 serving (without crust): 31
Carbohydrates, 1 serving (without crust): 6

Lemon Meringue Pie #1

9 in.	baked pie shell	23 cm
¾ c.	granulated fructose	190 mL
1½ c.	water	375 mL
¼ t.	salt	1 mL
½ c.	cornstarch	125 mL
¼ c.	cold water	60 mL
4	egg yolks, slightly beaten	4
½ c.	freshly squeezed lemon juice	125 mL
3 T.	low-calorie margarine	45 mL
1½ t.	grated fresh lemon peel	7 mL
4	egg whites	4
dash	salt	dash
¼ c.	granulated sugar replacement	60 mL

Combine fructose, the 1½-c. (375-mL) water, and salt in a medium-size, heavy saucepan. Heat to boiling. Combine cornstarch and the ¼-c.

(60-mL) cold water, stirring to blend thoroughly. Add to boiling mixture, stirring constantly. Cook and stir until mixture is clear and thickened. Remove from heat. Beat egg yolks and lemon juice together. Slowly stir into hot mixture. Return to heat and cook until mixture begins to boil. Stir in margarine and lemon peel. Cover and cool to room temperature. Beat egg whites and salt together until soft peaks form. Gradually add sugar replacement. Beat just until peaks are stiff. Pour lemon mixture into pie shell. Top with egg whites, sealing edges. Bake at 350 °F (175 °C) until peaks begin to brown.

Yield: 8 servings
Exchange, 1 serving (without crust): ½ medium-fat meat, ⅓ fruit
Calories, 1 serving (without crust): 88
Carbohydrates, 1 serving (without crust): 6

Lemon Meringue Pie #2

9 in.	baked pie shell	23 cm
1¼ c.	granulated sugar replacement	310 mL
7 T.	cornstarch	105 mL
¼ t.	salt	1 mL
1½ c.	water	375 mL
3	egg yolks, beaten	3
1 T.	low-calorie margarine	15 mL
1 t.	grated lemon peel	5 mL
½ c.	lemon juice	125 mL
1 recipe	Three Egg-Whites Meringue	1 recipe

Combine sugar replacement, cornstarch, salt, and water in a heavy saucepan. Stir to blend. Cook and stir over medium heat until mixture is clear and thickened. Remove from heat. Stir small amount of hot mixture into egg yolks; then return to saucepan. Cook and stir 2 to 3 minutes longer. Remove from heat and stir in margarine, lemon peel, and lemon juice. Cool slightly. Transfer to baked pie shell. Top with Three Egg-Whites Meringue (page 144), sealing edges. Bake at 350 °F (175 °C) for 7 to 10 minutes or until peaks begin to brown.

Yield: 8 servings
Exchange, 1 serving (without crust): ¾ medium-fat meat
Calories, 1 serving (without crust): 42
Carbohydrates, 1 serving (without crust): 3

Lime Pie

9 in.	baked pie shell	23 cm
1 c.	sorbitol	250 mL
⅓ c.	cornstarch	90 mL
¼ t.	salt	1 mL
1½ c.	water	375 mL
3	egg yolks, beaten	3
¼ c.	freshly squeezed lime juice	60 mL
1 T.	grated fresh lime zest	15 mL
	green food coloring (optional)	
1 recipe	Three Egg-Whites Meringue	1 recipe

Combine sorbitol, cornstarch, and salt in heavy saucepan. Stir to mix. Slowly stir water into mixture. Cook and stir over medium heat until mixture is clear and thickened. Remove from heat. Pour small amount of hot mixture into egg yolks; then return to saucepan. Bring to boil and cook for 1 minute. Remove from heat. Stir in lime juice and lime zest. Add green food coloring, if desired. Transfer immediately to baked pie shell. Top with Three Egg-Whites Meringue (page 144), sealing edges. Bake at 350 °F (175 °C) for 7 to 10 minutes or until peaks begin to brown.

Yield: 8 servings

Exchange, 1 serving (without crust): ½ medium-fat meat, 1 fruit

Calories, 1 serving (without crust): 103

Carbohydrates, 1 serving (without crust): 13

Open-Faced Green-Apple Pie

	baked pie shell	
6 c.	sliced green apples (peeled)	1500 mL
½ c.	apple juice	125 mL
3 T.	all-purpose four	45 mL
8 T.	prepared nondairy whipped topping	120 mL

Combine apples, apple juice, and flour in a nonstick saucepan. Cook and stir until thickened. Transfer to baked pie shell. Chill or serve warm with 1 T. (15 mL) of the nondairy whipped topping on each slice.

Yield: 8 servings

Exchange, 1 serving (without crust): 1⅓ fruits

Calories, 1 serving (without crust): 98

Carbohydrates, 1 serving (without crust): 22

Hot-Fudge Pie

9 in.	unbaked pie shell, chilled	23 cm
3 sq. (1 oz. each)	semi-sweet chocolate	3 sq. (30 g each)

⅓ c.	low-calorie margarine	90 mL
1 env.	butter-flavoring dry mix	1 env.
3	eggs, beaten	3
1 c.	sorbitol	250 mL
¼ c.	all-purpose flour	60 mL
2 t.	skim milk	10 mL
1 t.	vanilla extract	5 mL
dash	salt	dash

Combine chocolate and margarine in top of double boiler. Cook over boiling water until chocolate melts. Remove from heat and allow to cool to room temperature. Combine chocolate mixture, butter-flavoring mix, and eggs in large mixing bowl. Beat 10 to 15 minutes or until slightly thickened. Beat in sorbitol, flour, skim milk, vanilla, and salt. Transfer to unbaked pie shell. Bake at 375 °F (190 °C) for 35 to 40 minutes or until knife inserted in center comes out clean. Serve warm.

Yield: 8 servings
Exchange, 1 serving (without crust): ¾ fruit, ⅓ medium-fat meat, 1 fat
Calories, 1 serving (without crust): 189
Carbohydrates, 1 serving (without crust): 12

Chocolate-Chip Pie

9 in.	unbaked pie shell	23 cm
¼ c.	low-calorie margarine	60 mL
3	eggs, beaten	3
½ c.	liquid fructose	125 mL
¼ t.	salt	1 mL
1 t.	vanilla extract	5 mL
½ c.	chocolate chips	125 mL
¼ c.	chopped pecans	60 mL
2 T.	water	30 mL
2 t.	bourbon flavoring	10 mL

Cream margarine until light and fluffy. Beat in eggs, liquid fructose, salt, and vanilla. Continue beating 3 more minutes. Stir in chocolate chips, pecans, water, and bourbon flavoring. Transfer to unbaked pie shell. Bake at 375 °F (190 °C) for 35 to 40 minutes or until knife inserted in center comes out clean. Allow to cool.

Yield: 8 servings
Exchange, 1 serving (without crust): ½ fruit, ⅓ medium-fat meat, 1 fat
Calories, 1 serving (without crust): 162
Carbohydrates, 1 serving (without crust): 6

Cocoa Pie

9 in.	unbaked pie shell	23 cm
¾ c.	granulated fructose	190 mL
¼ c.	cocoa powder	60 mL
dash	salt	dash
2	eggs	2
¼ c.	low-calorie margarine	60 mL
15-oz. can	evaporated skim milk	427-g can
2 t.	vanilla extract	10 mL

Combine fructose, cocoa, and salt in a bowl, stirring to mix thoroughly. Combine eggs, margarine, evaporated milk, and vanilla in a mixing bowl; then beat to blend. Add cocoa mixture in small amounts, beating well after each addition. Transfer to unbaked pie shell. Bake at 350 °F (175 °C) for 45 to 50 minutes or until knife inserted in center comes out clean. Cool before serving.

Yield: 8 servings
Exchange, 1 serving (without crust): ¾ fruit, ¼ medium-fat meat, ½ fat
Calories, 1 serving (without crust): 162
Carbohydrates, 1 serving (without crust): 13

Lemon-Custard Pie

8 in.	unbaked pie shell, chilled	20 cm
3	eggs	3
¾ c.	water	190 mL
½ c.	granulated fructose	125 mL
⅓ c.	lemon juice	90 mL
1 t.	grated lemon zest	5 mL
dash	salt	dash

Combine eggs, water, fructose, lemon juice, lemon zest, and salt in a bowl. Beat to blend. Place chilled pie shell on shelf in oven, and pour custard into pie shell. Bake at 425 °F (220 °C) for 20 minutes; then reduce heat to 250 °F (120 °C) and bake 10 minutes more or until knife inserted in center comes out clean. Cool to room temperature.

Yield: 8 servings
Exchange, 1 serving (without crust): 1 fruit
Calories, 1 serving (without crust): 71
Carbohydrates, 1 serving (without crust): 13

Tarts

Lemon Tarts

10	prepared tart shells	10
½ c.	granulated fructose	125 mL
2 T.	low-calorie margarine	30 mL
1 t.	butter flavoring	5 mL
¼ c.	lemon juice	60 mL
1 t.	grated lemon zest	5 mL
1	egg, beaten	1

Combine fructose, margarine, butter flavoring, lemon juice, lemon zest, and egg in top of double boiler. Stir to mix. Cook and stir over hot water until mixture thickens. Pour into the 10 tart shells. Chill until firm.

Yield: 10 servings
Exchange, 1 serving (without crust): ½ fruit
Calories, 1 serving (without crust): 31
Carbohydrates, 1 serving (without crust): 5

Apricot Tarts

12	prepared tart shells	12
1½ c.	fresh apricots, cut in eighths	375 mL
2 t.	lemon juice	10 mL
2 drops	almond extract	2 drops
12 T.	prepared nondairy whipped topping	180 mL

Combine apricots, lemon juice, and almond extract in a bowl. Toss to mix. Fold apricots into nondairy whipped topping. Divide mixture evenly between the 12 tart shells. Chill thoroughly before serving.

Yield: 12 servings
Exchange, 1 serving (without crust): ⅓ fruit
Calories, 1 serving (without crust): 25
Carbohydrates, 1 serving (without crust): 8

Tart-Cherry Tarts

4	baked tart shells	4
2 c.	frozen tart cherries	500 mL
⅔ c.	sorbitol	180 mL
¼ t.	lavender leaves	1 mL
2	cardamom pods	2
1 T.	cornstarch	15 mL

Allow cherries to thaw. Drain liquid into a 1-c. (250-mL) measuring cup, pressing cherries with back of spoon to extract juice. Add extra water, if juice does not measure 1 c. (250 mL). Reserve cherries. Pour juice into a saucepan; then add sorbitol. Stir to mix. Either in the palm of your hand or in a mortar, crush lavender leaves and cardamom seeds from pod. Add to juice with cornstarch. Stir to dissolve cornstarch. Cook and stir over medium heat until mixture becomes clear and thick. Allow to cool for 3 minutes. Pour two-thirds of the liquid over the cherries; then fold to blend. Divide cherry mixture evenly between the four tart shells. Pour remaining liquid over cherry mixture in tart shells. Chill until firm.

Yield: 4 servings
Exchange, 1 serving (without crust): 1 fruit
Calories, 1 serving (without crust): 57
Carbohydrates, 1 serving (without crust): 15

Strawberry Tarts

6	prepared tart shells	6
3 c.	fresh strawberries	750 mL
½ c.	apple juice	125 mL
2 t.	unflavored gelatin	10 mL
½ c.	prepared nondairy whipped topping	125 mL

Clean the strawberries and then slice them in half lengthwise. Combine apple juice and gelatin in saucepan. Allow gelatin to soften for 5 minutes. Bring to a boil. Remove from heat and allow mixture to cool and thicken. Divide the strawberries evenly between the six tart shells. Pour gelatin over the top. Chill until firm. Divide the nondairy whipped topping evenly among the strawberry tarts.

Yield: 6 servings
Exchange, 1 serving (without crust): ¾ fruit
Calories, 1 serving (without crust): 42
Carbohydrates, 1 serving (without crust): 12

Dried-Apricot and -Prune Tarts

10	unbaked tart shells	10
1 c.	dried prunes	250 mL
1 c.	dried apricots	250 mL
dash	salt	dash
1 t.	cinnamon	5 mL
¾ c.	prune liquid	190 mL

Place prunes in saucepan. Cover with water and boil for about 15 minutes. Drain, reserving liquid. Remove pits from prunes; then cut them in half and place them back in saucepan. Rinse apricots (do not cook). Cut apricots in half and add to prunes. Next, add salt, cinnamon, and ¾ c. (190 mL) of the reserved prune liquid. If the liquid drained from the prunes does not measure ¾ c. (190 mL), add water to liquid. Bring to a boil; then reduce heat and cook until mixture thickens. Divide mixture evenly between the 10 tart shells. Bake at 425 °F (220 °C) for 15 minutes.

Yield: 10 servings
Exchange, 1 serving (without crust): 1 fruit
Calories, 1 serving (without crust): 56
Carbohydrates, 1 serving (without crust): 15

Currant Tartlets

18	unbaked tartlets	18
⅓ c.	dried currants	90 mL
1 t.	low-calorie margarine	5 mL
⅓ c.	granulated brown-sugar replacement	90 mL
1	egg white, slightly beaten	1
¼ t.	vanilla extract	1 mL

Wash currants and then cover with boiling water. Allow to soften for 5 minutes and then drain. While still hot, stir in margarine, brown-sugar replacement, egg white, and vanilla. Divide mixture evenly among the 18 tartlets. Cover tartlets loosely with aluminum foil. Bake at 350 °F (175 °C) for 15 minutes; then remove aluminum foil, reduce heat to 300 °F (150 °C), and cook for 10 more minutes.

Yield: 18 tartlets
Exchange, 2 tartlets (without crust): ⅓ fruit
Calories, 2 tartlets (without crust): 17
Carbohydrates, 2 tartlets (without crust): 4

Raspberry Cranberry Tarts

10	unbaked tart shells	10
10-oz. pkg.	frozen unsweetened raspberries	289-g pkg.
3 c.	fresh cranberries	750 mL
1 c.	granulated sugar replacement	250 mL
3 T.	cornstarch	45 mL
dash	salt	dash
3 T.	cold water	45 mL

Allow raspberries to thaw. Drain juice from raspberries by lightly pressing them with the back of a spoon into a 1-c. (250-mL) measuring cup. If juice does not measure 1 c. (250 mL), add water. Set raspberries aside. Combine the 1 c. (250 mL) of raspberry juice and the cranberries in a saucepan. Cook and stir over medium heat until cranberries begin to "pop." Remove from heat. Combine sugar replacement, cornstarch, and salt in a small mixing bowl. Stir in cold water to dissolve cornstarch; then add to cranberry mixture. Return to heat and cook until thickened. Remove from heat, and allow to cool for 5 minutes. Now stir in raspberries. Divide mixture evenly among the 10 tart shells. Bake at 400 °F (200 °C) for 10 to 15 minutes.

Yield: 10 servings
Exchange, 1 serving (without crust): ⅔ fruit
Calories, 1 serving (without crust): 40
Carbohydrates, 1 serving (without crust): 9

Date Tarts

8	prepared tart shells	8
2 c.	pitted dates	500 mL
1 c.	water	250 mL
2 T.	orange juice	30 mL

Combine dates and water in a saucepan; then cook to a thick paste. Remove from heat, and add orange juice. Allow mixture to cool. Divide mixture evenly among the eight tart shells.

Yield: 8 servings
Exchange, 1 serving (without crust): 1 fruit
Calories, 1 serving (without crust): 62
Carbohydrates, 1 serving (without crust): 16

Raisin Tarts ✓

8	frozen unbaked tart shells	8
1½ c.	raisins	375 mL
2 T.	chopped pecans	30 mL
1 T.	lemon juice	15 mL

Line tart pans as described on tart-shell package. Cover raisins with water; then bring to a boil. Allow to completely cool. Drain thoroughly. Combine drained raisins, pecans, and lemon juice in bowl. Mix. Fill tart shells. Bake at 400 °F (200 °C) for 15 to 20 minutes.

Yield: 8 servings
Exchange, 1 serving: 1 starch/bread, 1⅓ fruit, 1 fat
Calories, 1 serving: 203
Carbohydrates, 1 serving: 33

Strawberry Chiffon Tarts

12	prepared tart shells	12
2 c.	strawberries	500 mL
1 env.*	low-calorie strawberry-flavored gelatin	1 env.*
¼ c.	cold water	60 mL
½ c.	boiling water	125 mL
dash	salt	dash
1 c.	prepared nondairy whipped topping	250 mL
2	egg whites, stiffly beaten	2
12 whole	strawberries	12 whole

*four-servings size

Crush the 2 c. (500 mL) of strawberries. Set aside. Soften strawberry gelatin in cold water for 5 minutes. Add boiling water and then stir to dissolve gelatin. Stir in salt. Allow to cool to room temperature, but do not allow to set. Fold in the crushed strawberries. Cool until mixture is soft but no longer runny. Fold nondairy whipped topping and beaten egg whites into strawberry gelatin. (If mixture is too soft, chill until it holds a soft shape.) Divide mixture evenly among the 12 tart shells. Chill thoroughly. Just before serving, top each tart with a whole strawberry.

Yield: 12 servings
Exchange, 1 serving (without crust): ⅓ fruit
Calories, 1 serving (without crust): 20
Carbohydrates, 1 serving (without crust): 5

Strawberry Cheese Tarts

10	prepared tart shells	10
3 oz.	cream cheese	90 g
¼ c.	half-and-half	60 mL
3 T.	granulated sugar replacement	45 mL
2 c.	sliced fresh strawberries	500 mL
10 T.	prepared nondairy whipped topping	150 mL

Beat cream cheese and half-and-half together until stiff and smooth. With the back of a spoon or a small knife, line the tart shell with the cream-cheese mixture. Combine sugar replacement and strawberries in a bowl. Toss to mix. Divide the strawberries evenly among the 10 tart shells. Top each tart with 1 T. (15 mL) of nondairy whipped topping.

Yield: 10 servings
Exchange, 1 serving (without crust): ¼ fruit, ⅔ fat
Calories, 1 serving (without crust): 51
Carbohydrates, 1 serving (without crust): 3

Pumpkin Chiffon Tarts

12	prepared tart shells	12
1 env.	unflavored gelatin	1 env.
⅔ c.	granulated brown-sugar replacement	180 mL
1 t.	pumpkin-pie spice	5 mL
3	egg yolks, slightly beaten	3
⅔ c.	skim milk	180 mL
1 c.	canned pumpkin	250 mL
3	egg whites, stiffly beaten	3

Combine gelatin, brown-sugar replacement, and pie spice in a saucepan. Combine egg yolks and milk, mixing to blend. Pour into the saucepan. Stir to blend mixture. Allow gelatin to soften for 5 minutes. Bring mixture to boiling; then remove from heat and stir in canned pumpkin. Allow to cool until mixture holds a soft shape (do not allow to set). Fold in stiffly beaten egg whites. Divide mixture evenly among the 12 tart shells. Chill thoroughly before serving.

Yield: 10 servings
Exchange, 1 serving (without crust): ⅓ fruit
Calories, 1 serving (without crust): 19
ydrates, 1 serving (without crust): 3

Pineapple Tarts

	unbaked double crust	
2 c.	canned crushed pineapple, in its own juice, but drained	500 mL
2 T.	juice from crushed pineapple	30 mL
¼ c.	fresh sweet cherries	60 mL
¼ t.	grated lemon rind	1 mL

Roll out dough into a square. Cut into eight 5-in. (12-cm) squares. Arrange dough squares in muffin pans. Combine remaining ingredients in a bowl. Divide mixture evenly among the dough squares. Draw the corners of the squares together over the filling; then pinch the edges together. Bake at 425 °F (220 °C) for 20 to 25 minutes or until golden brown.

Yield: 8 servings
Exchange, 1 serving (without crust): ½ fruit
Calories, 1 serving (without crust): 27
Carbohydrates, 1 serving (without crust): 7

Raisin Nut Tarts

8	unbaked tart shells	8
⅓ c.	low-calorie margarine	90 mL
½ c.	granulated sugar replacement	125 mL
3	egg yolks, beaten	3
1	egg white, stiffly beaten	1
1 c.	chopped raisins	250 mL
1 c.	chopped walnuts	250 mL
1 t.	vanilla extract	5 mL

Cream margarine and sugar replacement together. Beat in egg yolks. Fold in stiffly beaten egg white. Next, add raisins, walnuts, and vanilla. Divide evenly between the eight tart shells. Bake at 350 °F (175 °C) for 10 to 15 minutes or until tops become slightly browned.

Yield: 8 servings
Exchange, 1 serving (without crust): 1 fruit, 1⅓ fat
Calories, 1 serving (without crust): 199
Carbohydrates, 1 serving (without crust): 14

Fruit Fried Tarts

2 T.	cold butter	30 mL
1 c.	sifted all-purpose flour	250 mL
1	egg yolk	1
3 T.	hot skim milk	45 mL
9 T.	puréed baby-food fruit	135 mL

Cut butter into flour. Blend egg yolk and milk together; then add to flour mixture. Knead well to make a smooth dough. Roll out to ⅛-in. (4-mm) thickness. Cut into six pastry rounds. Place 1½ T. (21 mL) of puréed fruit in center of each round. Fold over turnover-style and seal or pinch edges securely. Fry in hot fat at 365 °F (180 °C) until brown.

Yield: 6 servings
Exchange, 1 serving: 1¼ starch/bread, 1 fat
Calories, 1 serving: 132
Carbohydrates, 1 serving: 16

Fried Cream Tarts

Filling

1 c.	skim milk	250 mL
2 T.	granulated fructose	30 mL
dash	salt	dash
1 t.	low-calorie margarine	5 mL
4 t.	cornstarch	20 mL
4 t.	cold water	20 mL
2	egg yolks, beaten	2
1 t.	vanilla extract	5 mL

Combine skim milk, fructose, salt, and margarine in a saucepan. Heat to boiling. Dissolve cornstarch in the cold water. Stir into hot mixture. Cook and stir until mixture thickens. Remove from heat and slowly add small amount of hot mixture to egg yolks; then return to saucepan. Add vanilla and cook 5 minutes more. Cool thoroughly.

Crust

| 2 T. | cold butter | 30 mL |
| 1 c. | sifted all-purpose flour | 250 mL |

1	egg yolk	1
3 T.	hot skim milk	45 mL

Cut butter into flour. Blend egg yolk and milk together; then add to flour mixture. Knead well to make a smooth dough. Roll out to ⅛-in. (4-mm) thickness. Cut into six pastry rounds. Place 1 T. (15 mL) of filling in center of each round. Fold over turnover-style and seal or pinch edges securely. Fry in hot fat at 365 °F (180 °C) until brown.

Yield: 6 servings
Exchange, 1 serving: 1 low-fat milk, 1 fat, 1 bread
Calories, 1 serving: 205
Carbohydrates, 1 serving: 47

Tortes

Chocolate Chocolate Torte

8 oz.	sugar-free chocolate cake mix	227 g
1 pkg.*	sugar-free chocolate-fudge instant pudding and pie filling	1 pkg.*
2 c.	skim milk	500 mL
2 c.	prepared nondairy whipped topping	500 mL
⅓ c.	chopped walnuts	90 mL

*four-servings size

Bake cake as directed on package. Cool completely. Cut in half horizontally. Combine pudding mix and skim milk in a bowl. Beat for 1 or 2 minutes; then allow to set completely. Place bottom of cake on serving dish. Combine one-half of the pudding with one-third of the nondairy whipped topping. Fold to completely blend. Frost bottom half of cake with mixture. Sprinkle with one-third of the chopped walnuts. Chill thoroughly. Place remaining half of cake (top half) on frosted bottom half. Spread remaining pudding over top of cake, allowing to run slightly down the sides. Chill thoroughly. Frost or dot with remaining nondairy whipped topping. Sprinkle with remaining walnuts.

Yield: 10 servings
Exchange, 1 serving: 1⅔ starch/bread, 1 fat
Calories, 1 serving: 141
Carbohydrates, 1 serving: 27

Ice-Cream Sundae Torte

| 8 oz. | sugar-free chocolate cake mix | 227 g |
| 3 c. | peppermint ice cream | 750 mL |

| 2 c. | prepared nondairy whipped topping | 500 mL |
| ⅓ c. | chocolate chips, melted | 90 mL |

Bake cake as directed on package. Cool completely. Cut in half horizontally. Wrap each half in plastic wrap and freeze completely. Slightly soften ice cream. Spread ice cream evenly between the two halves. Wrap separately and freeze. Unwrap and stack layers. Frost top and sides with nondairy whipped topping. Then sprinkle with chocolate chips. Freeze. Allow 10 to 15 minutes of thawing time before serving.

Yield: 10 servings
Exchange, 1 serving: 2 starch/bread, 1 fat
Calories, 1 serving: 199
Carbohydrates, 1 serving: 21

Rum Torte

8 oz.	sugar-free white cake mix	227 g
⅓ c.	water	90 mL
⅓ c.	dark Jamaican rum	90 mL
1	egg white	1
¼ c.	skim milk	60 mL
2 T.	dark Jamaican rum	30 mL
1 pkg.	Estee 4-in-1 Frosting Mix	1 pkg.
1 T.	margarine	15 mL
1 c.	prepared nondairy whipped topping	250 mL

Combine cake mix, water, the ⅓-c. (90-mL) rum, and the egg white in a bowl. Beat for 4 or 5 minutes. Transfer to 8-in. (20-cm) round, lightly greased cake pan. Bake at 350 °F (175 °C) for 20 to 25 minutes. Allow cake to cool and then remove from pan. Cut cake horizontally into two layers. Now combine milk and the 2-T. (30-mL) rum in a saucepan. Over medium heat, gradually add frosting mix. Stir constantly until mixture becomes very thick. Remove from heat and stir in margarine. Allow to cool. Spread a thin coat of frosting and a thin coat of nondairy whipped topping on the bottom layer of the cake. Place top layer of cake on top. Spread with remaining frosting and whipped topping. Chill thoroughly before serving.
the cake layer. Place top layer of cake top. Spread with remaining

Yield: 12 servings
Exchange, 1 serving: 2 starch/bread, 1 fat
Calories, 1 serving: 175
Carbohydrates, 1 serving: 31

Coconut Chocolate Cream Torte

8 oz.	sugar-free chocolate cake mix	227 g
½ c.	unsweetened grated coconut	125 mL
1 c.	prepared nondairy whipped topping	250 mL
⅓ c.	semi-sweet chocolate chips	90 mL

Combine cake mix and ¼ c. (60 mL) of the coconut in a mixing bowl. Prepare cake as directed on package. Allow cake to cool completely. Cut cake in half horizontally. Spread nondairy whipped topping between layers. Melt chocolate chips over simmering water. Pour and spread melted chocolate over top of cake. Then sprinkle with remaining grated coconut.

Yield: 10 servings
Exchange, 1 serving: 1 starch/bread, 1 fat
Calories, 1 serving: 141
Carbohydrates, 1 serving: 21

Lemon Pistachio Torte

8 oz.	sugar-free white cake mix	227 g
1 T.	grated lemon zest	15 mL
1 t.	lemon flavoring	5 mL
1 pkg.*	sugar-free pistachio instant pudding and pie filling	1 pkg.*

*four-servings size

Mix cake as directed on package. Beat in lemon zest and lemon flavoring. Bake as directed on package. Cool completely. Cut cake in half horizontally. Chill. Prepare pistachio pudding with 2% low-fat milk as directed on package. Cool completely. Frost layers of cake with pistachio pudding. Chill thoroughly before serving.

Yield: 10 servings
Exchange, 1 serving: 1 starch/bread, 1 fat
Calories, 1 serving: 136
Carbohydrates, 1 serving: 24

Chantilly Strawberry Torte

¼ c.	Estee 4-in-1 Frosting Mix	60 mL
1 env.	nondairy whipped-topping mix	1 env.
½ c.	skim milk	125 mL

| 8 oz. | sugar-free white cake mix | 227 g |
| 1 c. | fresh strawberries | 250 mL |

Combine frosting mix, nondairy whipped-topping mix, and skim milk in a mixing bowl. With a fork, stir to blend. Place beaters in the bowl and refrigerate for at least an hour. Bake cake in 8-in. (20-cm) round pan as directed on package. Allow cake to cool completely. Slice strawberries lengthwise. Reserve 10 halves for top decoration. Cut cake horizontally into two layers. Beat frosting mix for 5 to 6 minutes or until it's thick and creamy. Spoon half of frosting mix over the bottom layer of cake. Place cut strawberries on top of frosting. Place top layer of cake on top. Spoon remaining frosting on top and decorate with reserved strawberry halves. Place in freezer. Chill or freeze. If frozen, thaw for 10 minutes before serving.

Yield: 10 servings
Exchange, 1 serving: 2 starch/bread, 1 fat
Calories, 1 serving: 165
Carbohydrates, 1 serving: 29

Duchess Torte

1 loaf	angel food cake, ready-made	1 loaf
1 pkg.	Estee 4-in-1 Frosting Mix	1 pkg.
1 t.	cherry flavoring	5 mL
2 c.	prepared nondairy whipped topping	500 mL
1 c.	pitted dark cherries	250 mL
¼ c.	crushed pineapple, well drained	60 mL
¼ c.	chopped almonds	60 mL

Slice cake into four layers. Prepare frosting mix as directed on package, adding the 1-t. (5-mL) cherry flavoring. Allow frosting to cool. Beat cooled frosting slightly to loosen. Gently fold frosting into the nondairy whipped topping. Reserve ½ c. (125 mL) of the frosting-topping mixture for top of cake. Quarter cherries; then set aside 6 to 10 for top decoration. Fold remaining cherries and the pineapple and almonds into non-reserved frosting-topping mixture. Fill layers. Spread top of cake with reserved frosting; then decorate with reserved cherries. Refrigerate.

Yield: 12 servings
Exchange, 1 serving: 1¾ starch/bread, 1 fat
Calories, 1 serving: 172
Carbohydrates, 1 serving: 30

Raspberry Torte

8 oz.	sugar-free white cake mix	227 g
2 t.	lemon flavoring	10 mL
1 c.	fresh raspberries	250 mL
¾ c.	prepared nondairy whipped topping	190 mL

Mix cake mix and lemon flavoring together. Prepare cake mix as directed on package. Allow cake to cool completely. Cut cake in half horizontally. Fold raspberries into whipped topping. Spread between layers and on top of cake. Chill thoroughly before serving.

Yield: 10 servings
Exchange, 1 serving: 1 starch/bread, 1 fat
Calories, 1 serving: 115
Carbohydrates, 1 serving: 19

Festive Cranberry Torte

2 c.	crushed fresh cranberries	500 mL
2 T.	grated orange peel	30 mL
½ c.	granulated fructose	125 mL
1 loaf	angel food cake, ready-made	1 loaf
3 c.	prepared nondairy whipped topping	750 mL

Combine cranberries, orange peel, and fructose in a saucepan. Stir to mix. Cook over low heat just until boiling. Cool completely. Slice angel food cake loaf into four layers. Spread one-fourth of the nondairy whipped topping on each layer. Spoon one-fourth of the chilled cranberries over the whipped topping. With a spoon or knife, gently swirl the cranberries into the whipped topping. Stack the layers. Refrigerate 2 to 3 hours before serving.

Yield: 12 servings
Exchange, 1 serving: 2 starch/bread, ¼ fruit
Calories, 1 serving: 172
Carbohydrates, 1 serving: 33

Graham-Cracker Cake Torte

1 c.	graham-cracker crumbs	250 mL
¼ c.	chopped walnuts	60 mL
2 T.	granulated sugar replacement	30 mL
2 T.	granulated fructose	30 mL
1 t.	cinnamon	5 mL

¼ c.	low-calorie margarine, melted	60 mL
8 oz.	sugar-free white cake mix	227 g
⅓ c.	semi-sweet chocolate chips, melted	90 mL

Mix graham-cracker crumbs, walnuts, sugar replacement, fructose, and cinnamon in a bowl. Pour melted margarine over the top of the mixture. Toss to mix. Press half of the mixture into the bottom of an 8-in. (20-cm)-square pan. Prepare cake mix as directed on package. Pour half of the cake batter over the crumb mixture in the bottom of the pan. Sprinkle with half of the remaining crumb mixture. Pour remaining batter over crumbs in pan. Sprinkle with remaining crumb mixture. Bake at 350 °F (175 °C) for 25 to 30 minutes or until torte tests done. While hot, drizzle with melted chocolate chips.

Yield: 12 servings
Exchange, 1 serving: 2 starch/bread, 1 fat
Calories, 1 serving: 172
Carbohydrates, 1 serving: 31

Lemon Torte

1 (9 in.) recipe	Meringue Crust	1 (23 cm) recipe
4	egg yolks	4
¼ c.	granulated fructose	60 mL
⅛ t.	salt	½ mL
3 T.	grated lemon peel	45 mL
3 T.	lemon juice	45 mL
2 c.	prepared nondairy whipped topping	500 mL

Beat egg yolks in top part of double boiler until they are thick and lemon colored. Beat in fructose gradually. Add salt, 1 T. (15 mL) of the grated lemon peel, and the lemon juice. Cook and stir over simmering water until thick. Cool completely. Spread half of the nondairy whipped topping into the Meringue Crust (turn to page 136 for the recipe). Pour the cooled lemon filling over the whipped topping. Decorate top of torte with remaining whipped topping. Then sprinkle with remaining 2 T. (30 mL) of grated lemon peel.

Yield: 8 servings
Exchange, 1 serving: ¾ medium-fat meat, ¼ fruit
Calories, 1 serving: 85
Carbohydrates, 1 serving: 5

Blueberry Cream Torte

8 oz.	sugar-free white cake mix	227 g
1½ c.	fresh blueberries	375 mL
2 T.	granulated fructose	30 mL
1 env.	nondairy whipped-topping mix	1 env.
½ c.	cold water	125 mL

Prepare cake as directed on package in loaf pan. Allow cake to cool completely. Cut cake into 10 even slices. Line the bottom of an 8-in. (20-cm)-square cake pan with plastic wrap. Cover bottom of plastic-lined pan with five of the cake slices. Crush blueberries; then stir in fructose. Allow to sit at room temperature for 30 minutes. Spoon half of the blueberries over the cake in pan. Combine nondairy whipped-topping mix and water in a bowl. Stir to mix. Place beaters in the bowl and chill for 30 minutes. Beat until thick and creamy, but not into soft peaks. Spoon half of the whipped topping over the blueberries in the pan. Cover with remaining cake slices. Spoon remaining blueberries over cake. Beat remaining whipped topping to soft peaks; then spread it over blueberries. Chill thoroughly before serving.

Yield: 16 servings
Exchange, 1 serving: 1 starch/bread
Calories, 1 serving: 74
Carbohydrates, 1 serving: 13

Grand-Marnier Torte

	vegetable spray	
1 c.	low-calorie margarine	250 mL
⅔ c.	granulated fructose	180 mL
4	eggs	4
1 c.	sifted cornstarch	250 mL
1 c.	sifted all-purpose flour	250 mL
1 t.	baking powder	5 mL
2 T.	grated orange rind	30 mL
2 T.	Grand Marnier	30 mL
1 T.	vanilla extract	15 mL

Coat a 10-in. (25-cm) Bundt pan with vegetable spray and then set it aside. Cream margarine with fructose in a large bowl for about 10 minutes or until mixture is light and fluffy. Beat in one egg. Gradually add ½ c. (125 mL) of the cornstarch. Beat in second egg. Beat in ½ c. (125 mL) of the flour. Beat in third egg. Beat in remaining ½ c. (125 mL) of the cornstarch. Beat in fourth egg. Combine remaining flour and baking powder; then beat into flour mixture. Beat well. Add orange rind, Grand Marnier, and vanilla. Transfer to greased Bundt pan. Bake at 375 °F (190 °C) for 45 to 55 minutes or until torte tests done. Cool in pan.

Yield: 20 servings
Exchange, 1 serving: 1½ starch/bread
Calories, 1 serving: 119
Carbohydrates, 1 serving: 21

Vienna Torte

1 c.	graham-cracker crumbs	250 mL
¼ c.	grated almonds	60 mL
2 T.	granulated sugar replacement	30 mL
2 T.	granulated fructose	30 mL
2 t.	cocoa powder	10 mL
½ t.	cinnamon	2 mL
⅛ t.	cloves	½ mL
¼ c.	low-calorie margarine, melted	60 mL
1 qt.	fresh raspberries	1 L
2 T.	granulated fructose	30 mL
½ c.	water	125 mL
1 T.	cornstarch	15 mL

Mix graham-cracker crumbs, almonds, sugar replacement, 2-T. (30-mL) fructose, cocoa, cinnamon, and cloves in a bowl. Pour melted margarine over the top of the mixture. Toss to mix. Press mixture into the bottom and up the sides of a 9-in. (23-cm) springform pan. Chill. Combine raspberries and 2-T. (30-mL) fructose in a bowl. With a potato masher, mash slightly. Combine water and cornstarch in a saucepan, stirring to blend. Then stir in raspberries. Cook and stir over medium heat until mixture is clear and very thick. Cool slightly. Spread mixture on top of graham crust in pan. Bake at 325 °F (165 °C) for 20 to 30 minutes. Remove from oven and chill thoroughly. Carefully push bottom of pan up to remove torte.

Yield: 12 servings
Exchange, 1 serving: 1 starch/bread, ½ fat
Calories, 1 serving: 103
Carbohydrates, 1 serving: 17

Puddings

Blueberry Betty

¼ c.	low-calorie margarine	60 mL
2 T.	water	30 mL
2 c.	white bread cubes, cut in ½-in. (1.25-cm) cubes	500 mL
2 c.	blueberries	500 mL
4 t.	lemon juice	20 mL
¼ c.	granulated fructose	60 mL
8 T.	prepared nondairy whipped topping	120 mL

Melt margarine and then mix with water and bread cubes. Transfer one-third of the bread-cubes mixture to the bottom of a baking dish. Top with 1 c. (250 mL) of the blueberries. Sprinkle with half of the lemon juice and half of the fructose. Repeat these layers, ending with the bread cubes. Bake at 350 °F (175 °C) for 20 minutes. Top each serving with 1 T. (15 mL) of nondairy whipped topping.

Yield: 8 servings
Exchange, 1 serving: 1 fruit, 1 starch/bread
Calories, 1 serving: 131
Carbohydrates, 1 serving: 27

Maple Custard

3	eggs	3
½ c.	dietetic maple syrup	125 mL
2 t.	maple flavoring	10 mL
dash	salt	dash
2 c.	2% low-fat milk	500 mL

Beat eggs with maple syrup, flavoring, and salt until mixture becomes foamy and well blended. Scald the milk. Gradually beat milk into egg mixture. Transfer mixture to six custard cups. Place custard cups in a pan of hot water. Bake at 350 °F (175 °C) for 35 to 40 minutes. Custard is done when tip of a knife inserted in center comes out clean. Chill thoroughly before serving.

Yield: 6 servings
Exchange, 1 serving: ½ medium-fat meat, ½ low-fat milk
Calories, 1 serving: 92
Carbohydrates, 1 serving: 8

Fried Cream

3	egg yolks	3
½ c.	all-purpose flour	125 mL
1 T.	cornstarch	15 mL
dash	salt	dash
1 T.	granulated fructose	15 mL
1 c.	skim milk	250 mL
1 t.	vanilla extract	5 mL
1	egg	1
1 t.	water	5 mL
½ c.	fine cornflake crumbs	125 mL
½ t.	cinnamon	2 mL
	fat for frying	

Beat egg yolks until they are thick and lemon colored. Sift flour, cornstarch, and salt together. Stir in fructose. Add flour mixture alternately with milk to thickened egg yolks. Cook in the top of a double boiler over boiling water. Stir until mixture becomes thick and smooth. Stir in vanilla. Transfer custard to lightly greased 8-in. (20-cm)-square baking pan. Allow to cool. Refrigerate and chill thoroughly. Now beat egg and water together. Cut custard into 16 strips, each 4 ×1 in. (10 × 2.5 cm). Carefully dip strips into the beaten egg-water mixture. Combine cornflake crumbs and cinnamon. Lightly coat strips with crumbs. Refrigerate. Fry a few strips at a time in 2 in. (5 cm) of hot fat in a medium-size skillet. Serve hot.

Yield: 16 servings
Exchange, 1 serving: ½ starch/bread, ¼ fat
Calories, 1 serving: 50
Carbohydrates, 1 serving: 5

Maple Pudding

1 env.	unflavored gelatin	1 env.
2¼ c.	skim milk	560 mL
3	egg yolks	3
dash	salt	dash
¾ c.	dietetic maple syrup	190 mL
1 t.	vanilla extract	5 mL
3	egg whites, stiffly beaten	3

Soften gelatin in milk in the top of a double boiler. Place over hot water and heat to scalding. Beat egg yolks and salt together; then stir in maple syrup. Add egg-yolk mixture to milk. Cook and stir over simmering water until mixture begins to thicken. Remove from heat. Stir in vanilla. Cool slightly. Beat in stiffly beaten egg whites. Transfer to 12 pudding dishes. Chill until pudding becomes very firm.

Yield: 12 servings
Exchange, 1 serving: ½ low-fat milk
Calories, 1 serving: 48
Carbohydrates, 1 serving: 7

Apple Cream

5 large	cooking apples	5 large
¼ c.	granulated fructose	60 mL
½ c.	water	125 mL
1	egg	1
¼ c.	skim milk	60 mL
¼ c.	heavy cream	60 mL

Peel and core apples; then cut them into eighths. Combine apples, fructose, and water in a saucepan. Bring to a boil; then reduce heat and cover and simmer for 10 to 15 minutes or until apples become tender. Drain, reserving the liquid. Allow apples to cool slightly. Transfer apples to a lightly greased baking dish. Now beat egg, skim milk, and cream together. Stir in apple liquid. Pour cream mixture over apples in baking dish. Bake at 350 °F (175 °C) for 25 to 30 minutes or until set.

Yield: 10 servings
Exchange, 1 serving: ½ fruit, ⅓ low-fat milk
Calories, 1 serving: 78
Carbohydrates, 1 serving: 11

Apple Betty

2 c.	white bread crumbs	500 mL
2 T.	low-calorie margarine, melted	30 mL
¼ c.	granulated brown-sugar replacement	60 mL
¼ t.	cinnamon	1 mL
dash	salt	dash
2 c.	chopped apples	500 mL

Combine bread crumbs, margarine, brown-sugar replacement, cinnamon, and salt in a bowl. Toss to mix. Arrange layers of crumb mixture and apples alternately in eight lightly greased individual baking dishes. Bake at 375 °F (190 °C) for 25 to 30 minutes. Serve hot or cold.

Yield: 8 servings
Exchange, 1 serving: 1 starch/bread
Calories, 1 serving: 73
Carbohydrates, 1 serving: 15

Cinnamon-Apple Custard

3	eggs	3
dash	salt	dash
2 large	apples	2 large
2 t.	lemon juice	10 mL
2 t.	cinnamon	10 mL
½ t.	nutmeg	2 mL
2 c.	skim milk	500 mL
⅓ c.	granulated sugar replacement	90 mL
1 T.	granulated fructose	15 mL

Beat eggs with salt until foamy and well blended. Peel, core, and chop apples. Sprinkle with lemon juice, cinnamon, and nutmeg. Toss to completely mix. Scald the milk. Remove from heat and stir in sugar replacement and fructose. Gradually beat milk into egg mixture. Divide the apple mixture evenly among eight custard cups. Pour egg-milk mixture over the apple mixture. Place custard cups in a pan of hot water. Bake at 350 °F (175 °C) for 35 to 40 minutes. Custard is done when tip of a knife inserted in center comes out clean. Chill thoroughly before serving.

Yield: 8 servings
Exchange, 1 serving: ½ medium-fat meat, ½ fruit
Calories, 1 serving: 89
Carbohydrates, 1 serving: 7

Gelatins

Raspberry Dessert

½ c.	low-calorie margarine	125 mL
1 c.	all-purpose flour	250 mL
¼ c.	finely chopped almonds	60 mL
2 T.	granulated fructose	30 mL
1	egg white	1
¼ t.	cream of tartar	1 mL
1 T.	fructose	15 mL
2 pkgs.*	sugar-free raspberry gelatin	2 pkgs.*
2 c.	hot water	500 mL
12-oz. pkg.	frozen unsweetened raspberries	360-g pkg.

*four-servings size

Combine margarine, flour, chopped almonds, and fructose. Mix until thoroughly blended. Pat into the bottom of a 9-in. (23-cm)-square cake pan. Bake at 325 °F (165 °C) for 15 minutes. Remove from oven and allow to cool completely. Now beat egg white and cream of tartar together until soft peaks form. Gradually beat in fructose. Spread on top of crumb base in pan. Now combine gelatin and hot water. Stir to dissolve gelatin. Add frozen raspberries. Stir to blend thoroughly, making sure raspberries have thawed. When the mixture has thickened to the consistency of egg whites, pour over meringue in pan. Refrigerate until firm.

Yield: 10 servings
Exchange, 1 serving: ½ starch/bread, 1½ fat, ⅓ fruit
Calories, 1 serving: 132
Carbohydrates, 1 serving: 17

Simply Blueberry Dessert

15	graham crackers	15
1 T.	water	15 mL
2 env.	unflavored gelatin	2 env.
1 qt.	water	1 L
2 T.	granulated fructose	30 mL
1 qt.	fresh blueberries	1 L
2 c.	prepared nondairy whipped topping	500 mL

Crush graham crackers into fine crumbs. Combine crumbs and the 1-T. (15-mL) water. Toss to mix. Dampen the insides of 12 dessert glasses. Sprinkle half of the crumbs into the glasses, slightly coating the sides. Now sprinkle gelatin over the 1-qt. (1-L) water, allowing it to soften for 5 minutes. Heat to boiling, stirring to dissolve gelatin. Remove from heat; then stir in fructose and blueberries. When gelatin has set to the consistency of egg whites, gently pour mixture into glasses until they are half full. Sprinkle top of blueberry mixture in glasses with the remaining crumbs. Then pour remaining blueberry mixture into glasses, over crumbs. Refrigerate until firm. Top with nondairy whipped topping before serving.

Yield: 12 servings
Exchange, 1 serving: ⅔ fruit, ⅓ starch/bread
Calories, 1 serving: 91
Carbohydrates, 1 serving: 16

Raspberry Cream Dessert √

1 pkg.* (30 g)	sugar-free raspberry gelatin	1 pkg.*
¾ c.	hot water	190 mL
10-oz. pkg.	frozen unsweetened raspberries	300-g pkg.
1 c.	ice cream	250 mL

*four-servings size

Dissolve gelatin in hot water. Add frozen raspberries. Stir raspberries, gently breaking them apart. Add ice cream, stirring to completely blend. Transfer to six dessert dishes or a serving dish. Chill until firm.

Yield: 6 servings
Exchange, 1 serving: ¾ fruit, ½ starch/bread
Calories, 1 serving: 85
Carbohydrates, 1 serving: 17

Apricot Peanut-Butter Dessert

1 pkg.*	sugar-free lemon gelatin	1 pkg.*
2 c.	hot water	500 mL
16	apricot halves, in their own juice	16
⅓ c.	creamy peanut butter	90 mL
¼ c.	chopped dates	60 mL
2 T.	chopped walnuts	30 mL

*four-servings size

Dissolve gelatin in the hot water; then chill to the consistency of egg whites. Drain apricots. Combine peanut butter, dates, and walnuts. Mix well. Divide peanut-butter mixture evenly among the cavities of the apricots; then press halves together. Place an apricot into a mould or dessert dish. Fill mould or dessert dish with the lemon gelatin. Chill until firm.

Yield: 8 servings
Exchange, 1 serving: 1 fruit, 1 fat
Calories, 1 serving: 119
Carbohydrates, 1 serving: 15

Sparkling Fruit Dessert

1 pkg.*	sugar-free lime gelatin	1 pkg.*
2 c.	hot water	500 mL
1	orange	1
1 c.	pineapple chunks, in their own juice	250 mL
1 c.	peach slices, in their own juice	250 mL
16	seedless green grapes	16

*four-servings size

Dissolve lime gelatin in hot water. Chill until the consistency of egg whites. Peel and section orange, removing seeds and membrane. Drain pineapple and peaches thoroughly. Reserve four peach slices. Add orange sections, pineapple chunks, and remaining peach slices to gelatin. Transfer to a mould or eight dessert dishes. Chill until firm. Now cut reserved peach slices in half crosswise. Decorate each serving with a half peach slice and two grapes.

Yield: 8 servings
Exchange, 1 serving: ½ fruit
Calories, 1 serving: 25
Carbohydrates, 1 serving: 8

Black-Cherry Dessert

1 qt.	black cherries	1 L
2 c.	water	500 mL
1 pkg.*	sugar-free cherry gelatin	1 pkg.*
½ c.	chopped blanched almonds	125 mL
12 T.	prepared nondairy whipped topping	180 mL

*four-servings size

Pit black cherries. Combine cherries and water in a saucepan. Cook over low heat until cherries are just tender. Drain thoroughly, reserving liquid. Measure liquid and add enough water to make 2 c. (500 mL). Heat liquid to boiling. Remove from heat; then stir in gelatin. Stir to dissolve. Chill until mixture is the consistency of egg whites. Then fold in cooked cherries and almonds. Transfer to dessert dishes, mould, or serving dish. Chill until firm. Decorate with nondairy whipped topping before serving.

Yield: 6 servings
Exchange, 1 serving: ⅔ fruit, 1½ fat
Calories, 1 serving: 101
Carbohydrates, 1 serving: 10

Pineapple Smoothy

16-oz. can	crushed pineapple, in its own juice	459-g can
1 env.	unflavored gelatin	1 env.
½ c.	cold water	125 mL
1 small	apple, grated	1 small
¼ c.	chopped hazelnuts	60 ml

Combine crushed pineapple and unflavored gelatin in a saucepan. Allow gelatin to soften for 5 minutes. Bring to a boil, stirring to dissolve gelatin. Remove from heat. Stir in cold water. Chill until mixture is the consistency of egg whites. Stir in grated apple. Transfer to four dessert dishes. Sprinkle with hazelnuts. Chill until firm.

Yield: 4 servings
Exchange, 1 serving: ⅔ fruit, ⅓ fat
Calories, 1 serving: 77
Carbohydrates, 1 serving: 10

Peach-Yogurt Dessert

1 env.	unflavored gelatin	1 env.
1 c.	hot peach juice	250 mL
10-oz. pkg.	frozen unsweetened peach slices	300-g pkg.
8 oz.	vanilla yogurt	240 g

Dissolve gelatin in peach juice. Add frozen peaches. Stir peaches and allow them to thaw. Stir in yogurt. Transfer to six dessert dishes or a serving dish. Chill until firm.

Yield: 6 servings
Exchange, 1 serving: ½ fruit, ⅓ skim milk
Calories, 1 serving: 65
Carbohydrates, 1 serving: 11

Grape Supreme

2 c.	white-grape juice	500 mL
1 env.	unflavored gelatin	1 env.
1 c.	seedless white grapes	250 mL
1 c.	seedless red grapes	250 mL

Sprinkle gelatin over grape juice in a saucepan. Allow to soften for 5 minutes. Bring to a boil, stirring until gelatin is dissolved. Chill until the consistency of egg whites. Fold in grapes. (If grapes are large, just cut them in half.) Transfer to serving dish. Chill until firm.

Yield: 6 servings
Exchange, 1 serving: 1⅓ fruits
Calories, 1 serving: 78
Carbohydrates, 1 serving: 20

Sparkling Orange Dessert

1 env.	unflavored gelatin	1 env.
1½ c.	water	375 mL
1 env.	unsweetened orange-drink mix	1 env.
1 T.	granulated fructose	15 mL
1 c.	mandarin orange slices	250 mL

Sprinkle gelatin over water in a saucepan. Allow gelatin to soften for 5 minutes. Bring to a boil, stirring to dissolve gelatin. Remove from heat. While hot, stir in orange-drink mix and fructose. Chill until the consistency of egg whites. Stir in mandarin orange slices. Transfer to four dessert dishes. Chill until firm.

Yield: 4 servings
Exchange, 1 serving: ½ fruit
Calories, 1 serving: 37
Carbohydrates, 1 serving: 8

Lemon-Fluff Dessert

1 pkg.*	sugar-free lemon gelatin	1 pkg.*
2 c.	prepared nondairy whipped topping	500 mL
	sprigs of mint	

*four-servings size

Prepare lemon gelatin as directed on package. When the gelatin is firm, beat with an electric mixer. Then beat in nondairy whipped topping. Transfer to 10 dessert glasses or serving dishes. Chill until firm. Decorate with mint sprigs just before serving.

Yield: 10 servings
Exchange, 1 serving: negligible
Calories, 1 serving: negligible
Carbohydrates, 1 serving: negligible

Cocktail Sour-Cream Supreme

1 pkg.*	sugar-free lime gelatin	1 pkg.*
½ t.	salt	2 mL
2 c.	hot water	500 mL
½ c.	low-calorie salad dressing	125 mL
½ c.	low-calorie sour cream	125 mL
1-lb. can	fruit cocktail, in its own juice	457-g can

*four-servings size

Dissolve gelatin and salt in hot water. Stir in salad dressing and sour cream. Chill until the consistency of egg whites. Drain fruit cocktail thoroughly. Fold fruit cocktail into thickened gelatin mixture. Chill until firm.

Yield: 8 servings
Exchange, 1 serving: 1 fat, ¼ fruit
Calories, 1 serving: 56
Carbohydrates, 1 serving: 4

Cranberry Mellow Dessert

1 env.	unflavored gelatin	1 env.
2 c.	cranberry fruit cocktail	500 mL
1 c.	mandarin orange slices	250 mL
1 c.	mini-marshmallows	250 mL

Sprinkle gelatin over cranberry fruit cocktail in saucepan. Allow to soften for 5 minutes. Bring to boiling, stirring to dissolve gelatin. Chill until mixture is the consistency of egg whites. Then fold in orange slices and marshmallows. Transfer to serving dish. Chill until firm.

Yield: 8 servings
Exchange, 1 serving: 1 fruit
Calories, 1 serving: 50
Carbohydrates, 1 serving: 17

Chocolate Swirl   *mousse?*

1 env.	unflavored gelatin	1 env.
1½ c.	water	375 mL
2 sq. (1 oz. each)	semi-sweet chocolate	2 sq. (30 g each)
1 T.	chocolate flavoring	15 mL
2 t.	butter flavoring	10 mL
2 c.	prepared nondairy whipped topping	500 mL
6 t.	finely chopped walnuts	30 mL

Sprinkle gelatin over water in saucepan. Allow to soften for 5 minutes. Bring to a boil, stirring to dissolve gelatin. Remove from heat; then stir in chocolate flavoring, and butter flavoring. Stir until chocolate is melted. Chill until mixture is the consistency of egg whites. Then fold and swirl in nondairy whipped topping. Transfer to six dessert glasses. Sprinkle each glass of chocolate swirl with 1 t. (5 mL) of the chopped walnuts. Chill until firm.

Yield: 6 servings
Exchange, 1 serving: ⅔ starch/bread
Calories, 1 serving: 62
Carbohydrates, 1 serving: 10

Apple Cheese Dessert

| 1 env. | unflavored gelatin | 1 env. |
| 1 c. | water | 250 mL |

1 oz.	sharp Cheddar cheese, shredded	30 g
1 c.	apple juice	250 mL
1 c.	grated apples	250 mL
1 t.	lemon juice	5 mL
2 t.	granulated sugar replacement	10 mL
6 T.	prepared nondairy whipped topping	90 mL

Sprinkle gelatin over water in saucepan. Allow gelatin to soften for 5 minutes. Heat over medium heat until mixture is warm; then add cheese. Stir to dissolve gelatin and melt cheese. Remove from heat and stir in apple juice. Chill until the consistency of egg whites. Now combine grated apple, lemon juice, and sugar replacement in a bowl. Toss to mix. Stir into slightly thickened gelatin mixture. Transfer to six individual moulds. Chill until firm. Unmould and top with nondairy whipped topping.

Yield: 6 servings
Exchange, 1 serving: 1 fruit
Calories, 1 serving: 60
Carbohydrates, 1 serving: 15

Tart Lime Dessert

1 env.	unflavored gelatin	1 env.
1 c.	water	250 mL
6 oz.-can	frozen limeade	177-g can
1 env.	nondairy whipped-topping mix	1 env.

Sprinkle gelatin over water in a saucepan. Allow to soften for 5 minutes. Heat to boiling, stirring to dissolve gelatin. Remove from heat; then stir in limeade until thawed. Add extra water to make 2 c. (500 mL) of liquid. Allow to cool but not set. Meanwhile, chill a bowl and electric beaters. Measure ½ c. (125 mL) of the lime liquid into the chilled bowl; then add the nondairy whipped-topping mix. Beat until thoroughly mixed. Place in freezer of refrigerator, and chill thoroughly. Place remaining lime liquid in refrigerator to set. Beat lime-whipped topping mixture until stiff peaks form. (Rechill if necessary.) Fold set lime gelatin and lime-whipped topping mixture together. Transfer to serving dish.

Yield: 8 servings
Exchange, 1 serving: 1 fruit
Calories, 1 serving: 51
Carbohydrates, 1 serving: 13

Orange-Sherbet Dessert

1 pkg.*	sugar-free orange gelatin	1 pkg.*
½ c.	hot water	125 mL
2 c.	orange sherbet	500 mL

*four-servings size

Dissolve gelatin in hot water. Stir in orange sherbet until melted. Pour into four individual serving dishes. Chill until firm.

Yield: 4 servings
Exchange, 1 serving: 1 starch/bread
Calories, 1 serving: 96
Carbohydrates, 1 serving: 13

Peanut Butterscotch Delight

1 env.	unflavored gelatin	1 env.
1½ c.	water	375 mL
½ c.	chunky peanut butter	125 mL
1 pkg.*	sugar-free butterscotch instant pudding and pie filling	1 pkg.*

* four-servings size

Sprinkle gelatin over water in saucepan. Allow to soften for 5 minutes. Bring to a boil, stirring to dissolve gelatin. Remove from heat; then stir in peanut butter until melted. Chill until gelatin mixture is the consistency of egg whites. Chill until firm. Prepare pudding as directed on package. When both the gelatin and the pudding are firm, layer the pudding and the gelatin into eight dessert dishes, starting with pudding and ending with gelatin. Chill until firm.

Yield: 8 servings
Exchange, 1 serving: 1 starch/bread, 1 fat
Calories, 1 serving: 105
Carbohydrates, 1 serving: 13

Soufflés

Chocolate-Pudding Soufflé with Bananas

	vegetable spray	
½ c.	semi-sweet chocolate chips	125 mL
¼ c.	whipping cream	60 mL
1 t.	instant coffee, powder	5 mL
2	egg yolks	2
½ t.	cinnamon	2 mL
1 small	banana, sliced	1 small
3	egg whites	3
1 T.	granulated sugar replacement	15 mL

Using a vegetable spray, oil a shallow 4-c. (1000-mL) gratin pan or baking dish. Set aside. Combine chocolate chips, whipping cream, and instant coffee in the top of a double boiler. Heat and stir over simmering water until chips are melted and mixture is smooth. Remove pan from over water. Immediately beat in egg yolks and cinnamon. Lay banana slices on the bottom of the prepared shallow pan. Set aside. Beat egg whites until soft peaks form. Sprinkle sugar replacement over top of egg whites, beating until stiff but not dry. Fold one-fourth of the egg whites into the chocolate mixture to loosen. Then carefully fold remaining egg whites into chocolate mixture. Spread chocolate carefully over bananas in pan. Bake in a preheated 425 °F (220 °C) oven until chocolate mixture puffs and springs back when touched.

Yield: 8 servings
Exchange, 1 serving: ⅔ starch/bread, 1 fat
Calories, 1 serving: 110
Carbohydrates, 1 serving: 10

Grand-Marnier Soufflé

½ c.	skim milk	125 mL
½ c.	orange juice	125 mL
½ t.	vanilla extract	2 mL
1 T.	grated orange peel	15 mL
3	egg yolks, at room temperature	3
¼ c.	all-purpose flour	60 mL
1 T.	Grand Marnier	15 mL
5	egg whites, at room temperature	5 mL
pinch	cream of tartar	pinch
2 T.	granulated sugar replacement	30 mL

Combine milk, orange juice, vanilla, and orange peel in a heavy nonstick pan. Bring to a boil over medium heat and cook for 1 minute. Remove from heat and allow to cool slightly. Beat egg yolks and flour until blended. Add egg-yolk mixture to milk mixture, stirring to blend. Return to medium heat. Cook and stir until custard mixture becomes very thick. Remove from heat and allow to cool until barely warm to the touch. Generously grease a 6-c. (1500-mL) soufflé dish. Set aside. Stir Grand Marnier into custard mixture. Beat egg whites and cream of tartar together until soft peaks form. Sprinkle sugar replacement over egg whites, beating until stiff but not dry. Fold one-fourth of the stiffly beaten egg whites into the custard to loosen. Then fold in remaining egg whites. Pour mixture into prepared dish. Spread evenly. Bake at 400 °F (200 °C) for 20 to 25 minutes or until soufflé is puffy and firm to the touch.

Yield: 8 servings
Exchange, 1 serving: ½ skim milk
Calories, 1 serving: 59
Carbohydrates, 1 serving: 5

Black-Walnut Soufflé

6	egg yolks, at room temperature	6
¼ c.	granulated fructose	60 mL
¼ c.	granulated sugar replacement	60 mL
½ c.	ground black walnuts	125 mL
6	egg whites, at room temperature	6

Beat egg yolks until light; then add fructose and sugar replacement. Beat until thick and lemon colored. Add black walnuts. Beat egg whites until stiff but not dry. Fold egg-yolk mixture into egg whites. Pour into a 2- or 2½-qt. (2- or 2½-L) well greased baking dish. Set dish into pan of hot water. Bake at 325 °F (165 °C) for 60 to 65 minutes or until soufflé is firm.

Yield: 10 servings
Exchange, 1 serving: ⅓ starch/bread, 1 fat
Calories, 1 serving: 82
Carbohydrates, 1 serving: 5

Plain Sweet Soufflé

1 medium	vanilla bean	1 medium
1 c.	skim milk	250 mL
3	egg yolks, at room temperature	3
2 T.	granulated sugar replacement	30 mL
¼ c.	all-purpose flour	60 mL
5	egg whites, at room temperature	5
pinch	cream of tartar	pinch
1 T.	granulated sugar replacement	15 mL

Cut vanilla bean in half lengthwise. Bring milk and vanilla bean to a boil over medium heat in nonstick pan. Remove from heat. Cover and allow to steep for 30 minutes. Remove vanilla bean. (It may be rinsed and used for other dishes.) Return milk to heat and bring to a boil. Remove from heat. Beat egg yolks and the 2-T. (30-mL) sugar replacement in a bowl until creamy; then beat in flour just until mixed. Gradually whisk or beat into hot milk in pan. Return pan to medium heat. Cook and stir until custard becomes very thick. Remove from heat and allow to cool until warm to the touch. Generously grease a 6-c. (1500-mL) soufflé dish or casserole. Set aside. Beat egg whites and cream of tartar together until soft peaks form; then sprinkle the 1-T. (15-mL) sugar replacement over top of egg whites. Beat until stiff but not dry. Lightly beat custard until smooth. Fold half of egg-white mixture into custard to loosen. Then fold in remaining egg whites. Pour into prepared dish or casserole. Spread evenly. Bake at 400 °F (200 °C) for 20 to 25 minutes or until soufflé is puffy and firm to the touch.

Yield: 8 servings
Exchange, 1 serving: ½ skim milk, ⅓ fat
Calories, 1 serving: 57
Carbohydrates, 1 serving: 5

Almond Soufflé

1 c.	skim milk	250 mL
1	vanilla bean, split lengthwise	1
3	egg yolks, at room temperature	3
2 T.	granulated sugar replacement	30 mL
¼ c.	all-purpose flour	60 mL
⅓ c.	finely ground, toasted almonds	90 mL
5	egg whites, at room temperature	5
pinch	cream of tartar	pinch
4 t.	granulated sugar replacement	20 mL

Combine milk and vanilla bean in heavy nonstick pan. Bring to a boil over medium heat. Remove from heat, cover, and allow to steep for 30 minutes. Remove vanilla bean (it can be rinsed and saved for later use). Return milk to a boil. Remove from heat. Beat egg yolks and the 2-T. (30-mL) sugar replacement for 1 minute. Blend in flour. Return mixture to medium heat. Cook and stir until mixture becomes very thick. Remove from heat and blend in almonds. Allow to cool until warm to the touch. Now beat egg whites and cream of tartar together until soft peaks form. Gradually beat in the 4-t. (20-mL) sugar replacement until whites are stiff but not dry. Pour into eight individual, well greased custard cups. Bake at 400 °F (200 °C) for 12 to 15 minutes or until soufflé is puffed and almost firm to the touch.

Yield: 8 servings
Exchange, 1 serving: ½ skim milk, 1 fat
Calories, 1 serving: 91
Carbohydrates, 1 serving: 5

Blueberry Soufflé

1 c.	frozen blueberries, thawed	250 mL
½ c.	skim milk	125 mL
¼ c.	all-purpose flour	60 mL
2 T.	granulated fructose	30 mL
2 t.	low-calorie margarine	10 mL
3	egg whites	3
pinch	cream of tartar	pinch
	vegetable spray	

Combine blueberries, milk, flour, and fructose in a heavy nonstick saucepan. Cook and stir over medium heat until mixture becomes very thick. Remove from heat and stir in margarine. Allow to cool. Beat egg whites with cream of tartar until stiff but not dry. Fold one-fourth of the egg whites into the blueberry mixture to loosen. Then fold in remaining egg whites. Transfer to four vegetable-sprayed custard cups. Bake at 400 °F (200 °C) for 15 to 20 minutes or until soufflé is almost firm to the touch. Serve immediately.

Yield: 4 servings
Exchange, 1 serving: ½ fruit, ¾ starch/bread
Calories, 1 serving: 91
Carbohydrates, 1 serving: 17

Cappuccino Soufflé

1 c.	warm skim milk	250 mL
1 t.	vanilla extract	5 mL
5 t.	instant espresso, powder	25 mL
2 T.	boiling water	30 mL
3	egg yolks, at room temperature	3
3 T.	granulated sugar replacement	45 mL
¼ c.	all-purpose flour	60 mL
1 oz.	semi-sweet chocolate, finely ground	30 g
5	egg whites, at room temperature	5
pinch	cream of tartar	pinch

Combine milk and vanilla in medium-size, heavy saucepan. Heat to boiling. Allow to cool until warm to the touch. Dissolve espresso powder in the boiling water. Cool to room temperature. Beat egg yolks and granulated sugar replacement together until creamy. Then beat in flour. Slowly beat or whisk egg mixture into milk. Return to medium heat and whisk until custard thickens. Remove from heat and gradually whisk in chocolate and espresso. Cool to room temperature. Beat egg whites with cream of tartar until stiff but not dry. Fold one-fourth of egg whites into custard to loosen; then fold in remaining egg whites. Transfer to well greased 6-c. (1500-mL) soufflé dish or casserole. Bake at 400 °F (200 °C) for 20 to 25 minutes or until soufflé is firm to the touch.

Yield: 6 servings
Exchange, 1 serving: ½ starch/bread, ½ medium-fat meat, ½ fat
Calories, 1 serving: 110
Carbohydrates, 1 serving: 8

Lemon Soufflé

1 c.	water	250 mL
¼ c.	lemon juice	60 mL
¼ c.	granulated fructose	60 mL
1 t.	grated lemon peel	5 mL
¼ c.	all-purpose flour	60 mL
2	egg yolks, at room temperature	2
4	egg whites, at room temperature	4
pinch	cream of tartar	pinch
	vegetable spray	

Combine water, lemon juice, fructose, lemon peel, and flour in a heavy nonstick saucepan. Cook and stir over medium heat until custard thickens. Slightly beat egg yolks. Pour small amount of hot lemon custard into egg yolks, stirring to blend. Pour egg-yolk mixture into saucepan with custard. Cook and stir until thick. Remove from heat, cover, and allow to cool. Beat egg whites with cream of tartar until stiff but not dry. Fold one-fourth of egg whites into custard mixture to loosen. Then fold in remaining egg whites. Transfer to vegetable-sprayed 6-c. (1500-mL) soufflé pan. Bake at 400 °F (200 °C) for 25 to 30 minutes or until soufflé is almost firm. Serve immediately.

Yield: 8 servings
Exchange, 1 serving: 1 fruit, ½ medium-fat meat
Calories, 1 serving: 122
Carbohydrates, 1 serving: 18

Coconut Soufflé with Ginger

1 c.	2% low-fat milk	250 mL
3	egg yolks, at room temperature	3
2 T.	granulated sugar replacement	30 mL
¼ c.	all-purpose flour	60 mL
1 t.	vanilla extract	5 mL
½ c.	unsweetened flaked coconut	125 mL
1 T.	ginger	15 mL
5	egg whites, at room temperature	5
pinch	cream of tartar	pinch
2 T.	granulated sugar replacement	30 mL

Bring milk to a boil over medium heat in heavy nonstick pan. Beat egg yolks and sugar replacement together until creamy. Blend in flour and vanilla. Gradually beat milk into egg-yolk mixture. Return to medium heat. Cook and stir until custard becomes very thick. Remove custard from heat and allow to cool until barely warm to the touch. Stir or whisk custard until smooth. Blend in coconut and ginger. Beat egg whites with cream of tartar until soft peaks form. Sprinkle sugar replacement over egg whites, beating until stiff but not dry. Fold one-fourth of the egg whites into the custard mixture to loosen. Then fold in remaining egg whites. Transfer to a well greased 6-c. (1500-mL) soufflé dish or casserole. Spread evenly. Bake at 400 °F (200 °C) for 20 to 25 minutes or until soufflé is puffy and firm to the touch.

Yield: 8 servings
Exchange, 1 serving: ½ skim milk, 1 fat
Calories, 1 serving: 79
Carbohydrates, 1 serving: 5

Pineapple Soufflé

1 env.	unflavored gelatin	1 env.
¼ c.	cold water	60 mL
3	egg yolks	3
1 T.	lemon juice	15 mL
¼ c.	granulated fructose	60 mL
dash	salt	dash
⅔ c.	canned crushed pineapple, in its own juice, but drained	180 mL
½ c.	prepared nondairy whipped topping	125 mL
3	egg whites, stiffly beaten	3

Sprinkle gelatin over water in a bowl. Allow to soften for 5 minutes. Meanwhile, combine egg yolks, lemon juice, fructose, and salt in another bowl. Beat until blended. Transfer egg-yolk mixture to saucepan. Cook and stir over medium heat until mixture thickens. Add softened gelatin and stir until gelatin dissolves. Stir in pineapple. Remove from heat and allow to cool. When mixture is very thick and syrupy, fold in nondairy whipped topping and stiffly beaten egg whites. Transfer to a mould and chill thoroughly. When firm, unmould. If desired, decorate with lettuce leaves.

Yield: 10 servings
Exchange, 1 serving: ⅔ fruit, ½ fat
Calories, 1 serving: 70
Carbohydrates, 1 serving: 9

Pumpkin Soufflé

1 c.	skim milk	250 mL
3 T.	granulated fructose	45 mL
dash	salt	dash
3 T.	low-calorie margarine	45 mL
1 t.	nutmeg	5 mL
2 c.	mashed pumpkin	500 mL
2	egg yolks, slightly beaten	2
½ c.	raisins	125 mL
3	egg whites, stiffly beaten	3

Combine milk, fructose, salt, margarine, and nutmeg in a saucepan. Warm slightly to dissolve fructose. Remove from heat and add pumpkin. Beat until fluffy. Beat in egg yolks. Stir in raisins. Gently fold mixture into stiffly beaten egg whites. Transfer to 2- or 2½-qt. (2- or 2½-L) well greased baking dish. Bake at 350 °F (175 °C) for 50 to 60 minutes or until soufflé is firm.

Yield: 10 servings
Exchange, 1 serving: 1 fruit, ⅔ fat
Calories, 1 serving: 85
Carbohydrates, 1 serving: 12

Banana Soufflé

1 env.	unflavored gelatin	1 env.
¼ c.	cold water	60 mL
2	egg yolks	2
¼ c.	pineapple juice	60 mL
¼ c.	granulated sugar replacement	60 mL
½ t.	banana flavoring	2 mL
dash	salt	dash
1 c.	mashed bananas	250 mL
½ c.	prepared nondairy whipped topping	125 mL
3	egg whites, stiffly beaten	3

Sprinkle gelatin over water in a bowl. Allow to soften for 5 minutes. Meanwhile, combine egg yolks, pineapple juice, sugar replacement, banana flavoring, and salt in another bowl. Beat until blended. Transfer egg-yolk mixture to saucepan. Cook and stir over medium heat until mixture thickens. Add softened gelatin and stir until gelatin dissolves. Remove from heat. Stir in mashed bananas and allow to cool. When mixture is very thick and syrupy, fold in whipped topping and egg whites. Transfer to a mould or serving dish and chill thoroughly. When firm, unmould. If desired, decorate with lettuce leaves.

Yield: 10 servings
Exchange, 1 serving: ⅔ fruit, ½ fat
Calories, 1 serving: 65
Carbohydrates, 1 serving: 9

Strawberry Cream Soufflé

1 env.	unflavored gelatin	1 env.
¼ c.	granulated sugar replacement	60 mL
dash	salt	dash
2	egg yolks	2
¼ c.	water	60 mL
10-oz. pkg.	frozen unsweetened strawberries	289-g pkg.
1 T.	fresh lemon juice	15 mL
	red food coloring	
2	egg whites, stiffly beaten	2
2 c.	prepared nondairy whipped topping	500 mL

Mix gelatin, sugar replacement, and salt together in the top of a double boiler. Beat the egg yolks with the water; then add to gelatin mixture. Thaw and slice strawberries. Add strawberries to mixture. Cook and stir over simmering water until the gelatin thoroughly dissolves and the mixture thickens. Remove from heat and stir in lemon juice and food coloring. Chill to syrupy consistency. Fold gelatin mixture into stiffly beaten egg whites. Then, fold nondairy whipped topping into mixture. Transfer to a 5- to 6-c.(1250- to 1500-mL) mould. Chill until firm. Unmould onto chilled serving plate. Garnish with shredded lettuce, if desired.

Yield: 12 servings
Exchange, 1 serving: ⅔ fruit, ½ fat
Calories, 1 serving: 71
Carbohydrates, 1 serving: 10

Coffee Soufflé

1 env.	unflavored gelatin	1 env.
¼ c.	cold coffee	60 mL
⅔ c.	granulated fructose	180 mL
dash	salt	dash
1 c.	hot strong coffee	250 mL
5	egg yolks, slightly beaten	5
1 t.	vanilla extract	5 mL
5	egg whites, stiffly beaten	5
2 c.	prepared nondairy whipped topping	500 mL

Soften gelatin in cold coffee for 5 minutes. Add fructose, salt, and hot coffee to slightly beaten egg yolks. Transfer egg-yolk mixture to heavy nonstick saucepan. Cook and stir until mixture is slightly thickened. Remove from heat; then stir in softened gelatin and vanilla. Cool to syrupy consistency. Fold mixture into stiffly beaten egg whites, then into nondairy whipped topping. Transfer to a 1½- to 2-qt. (1½- to 2-L) mould or into 12 individual moulds. Chill until firm.

Yield: 12 servings
Exchange, 1 serving: ⅔ fruit, ½ high-fat meat
Calories, 1 serving: 96
Carbohydrates, 1 serving: 7

Lemon-Lovers' Soufflé

1 env.	unflavored gelatin	1 env.
1 c.	cold water	250 mL
⅓ c.	lemon juice	90 mL
1 T.	chopped fresh lemon peel	15 mL
1	egg yolk, slightly beaten	1
3 T.	xylitol	45 mL
3	egg whites, stiffly beaten	3
2 c.	prepared nondairy whipped topping	500 mL

Soften gelatin in cold water for 5 minutes in a heavy nonstick saucepan. Add lemon juice, lemon peel, slightly beaten egg yolk, and xylitol. Cook and stir over medium heat until mixture barely comes to a boil. Remove from heat and allow to cool until mixture is slightly thickened. Fold mixture into stiffly beaten egg whites and nondairy whipped topping. Transfer to a 6- to 7-c. (1500- to 1750-mL) mould. Chill until firm. Unmould onto chilled serving plate.

Yield: 12 servings
Exchange, 1 serving: ⅔ fruit, 1 fat
Calories, 1 serving: 76
Carbohydrates, 1 serving: 6

Sugar 'n' Spice Soufflé

1 env.	unflavored gelatin	1 env.
½ c.	cold water	125 mL
1¼ c.	water	310 mL
3 in.	cinnamon stick, broken into pieces	7.5 cm
¼ t.	nutmeg	1 mL
⅓ c.	granulated fructose	90 mL
2 T.	vanilla extract	30 mL
2	egg whites, stiffly beaten	2
1 c.	prepared nondairy whipped topping	250 mL

Sprinkle gelatin over the ½-c. (125-mL) cold water. Allow to soften for 5 minutes. Combine the 1¼-c. (310-mL) water, cinnamon-stick pieces, nutmeg, and fructose in a saucepan. Bring to a boil. Reduce heat and then cover and allow to simmer for 5 minutes. Remove from heat. Remove cinnamon pieces. Add softened gelatin and vanilla, stirring to dissolve gelatin completely. Allow to cool to slightly thickened stage, stirring occasionally to keep nutmeg in suspension. Fold into egg whites and whipped topping. Transfer to six individual moulds or custard cups. Chill until firm.

Yield: 12 servings
Exchange, 1 serving: ⅓ fruit, ⅓ fat
Calories, 1 serving: 42
Carbohydrates, 1 serving: 5

Cookies

Bachelor Buttons

¾ c.	low-calorie margarine	190 mL
½ c.	granulated brown-sugar replacement	125 mL
¼ c.	granulated sugar replacement	60 mL
¼ c.	liquid fructose	60 mL
1 T.	water	15 mL
1	egg	1
2 c.	all-purpose flour	500 mL
1 t.	baking soda	5 mL
¼ t. each	ginger, cinnamon, salt	1 mL each
1 t.	vanilla extract	5 mL
½ c.	chopped walnuts	125 mL

Cream together the margarine, both sugar replacements, fructose, and water until light and fluffy. Add egg and beat well. Combine flour, baking soda, ginger, cinnamon, and salt. Add to the creamed mixture and mix well. Next, stir in vanilla and nuts. Cover. Chill for several hours or overnight. Then form dough into 1-in. (2.5-cm) balls. Place on lightly greased cookie sheets about 2 in. (5 cm) apart. Gently press each cookie with a fork. Bake at 350 °F (175 °C) for 15 to 17 minutes. Allow cookies to cool slightly on cookie sheet before removing.

Yield: 42 cookies
Exchange, 1 cookie: ⅓ starch/bread, ½ fat
Calories, 1 cookie: 51
Carbohydrates, 1 cookie: 6

Cerealroons

3	egg whites, slightly beaten	3
½ t.	salt	2 mL

½ c.	granulated sugar replacement	125 mL
¼ c.	granulated fructose	60 mL
2 t.	liquid fructose	10 mL
¼ t.	almond extract	1 mL
2 c.	unsweetened cornflakes	500 mL
2 c.	unsweetened flaked coconut	500 mL

Beat egg whites with salt until foamy. Combine sugar replacement and granulated fructose in a bowl. Stir to mix. Add this sweetener, two tablespoons at a time, to the egg whites, beating well after each addition. Beat in liquid fructose and almond extract. Fold in cornflakes and coconut. Drop batter by teaspoonfuls onto an ungreased cookie sheet lined with brown paper. Then bake at 325 °F (165 °C) for 20 minutes.

Yield: 36 cookies
Exchange, 1 cookie: $^1/_5$ starch/bread
Calories, 1 cookie: 19
Carbohydrates, 1 cookie: 3

Oatmeal Coconut Cookies

2	eggs	2
¾ c.	granulated fructose	190 mL
1 c.	low-calorie margarine, melted	250 mL
1 c.	all-purpose flour	250 mL
1 t.	salt	5 mL
1 t.	baking powder	5 mL
1 t.	baking soda	5 mL
3 c.	quick-cooking oatmeal (uncooked)	750 mL
1 c.	unsweetened flaked coconut	250 mL

Beat eggs in a large mixing bowl. Add fructose and beat for 3 to 4 minutes. Slowly beat in melted margarine. Sift flour, salt, baking powder, and baking soda together. Beat into egg mixture. Add oatmeal and coconut; then beat until well blended. Allow to rest for 2 minutes. Drop batter by teaspoonfuls onto an ungreased cookie sheet. Bake at 350 °F (175 °C) for 12 to 14 minutes. Remove from cookie sheet; then move to rack to cool.

Yield: 72 cookies
Exchange, 1 cookie: ½ starch/bread
Calories, 1 cookie: 48
Carbohydrates, 1 cookie: 7

Melted-Chocolate Cookies

¾ c.	semi-sweet chocolate chips	190 mL
1½ c.	all-purpose flour	375 mL
1 t.	baking soda	5 mL
½ t.	salt	2 mL
½ c.	low-calorie margarine, softened	125 mL
⅓ c.	granulated fructose	90 mL
1 t.	vanilla extract	5 mL
1	egg	1

Melt chocolate chips in a microwave oven or over simmering water. Cool to room temperature. Combine flour, baking soda, and salt in a bowl. Stir to blend. In a medium-size mixing bowl, beat margarine and fructose until smooth. Beat in vanilla and egg. Continue beating at least 2 more minutes. Add melted chocolate chips and beat well. Then gradually beat in flour mixture. Drop batter by teaspoonfuls onto an ungreased cookie sheet. Bake at 375 °F (190 °C) for 8 minutes. (Cookies will be soft.) Allow to cool on pan for 2 to 3 minutes; then move to rack. These are crisp chocolate cookies. If you prefer softer cookies, try putting a slice of apple in your cookie tin with the baked cookies.

Yield: 48 cookies
Exchange, 1 cookie: ½ starch/bread
Calories, 1 cookie: 42
Carbohydrates, 1 cookie: 6

Bert's Oatmeal Bars

½ c.	low-calorie margarine	125 mL
½ c.	granulated fructose	125 mL
½ c.	water	125 mL
4 c.	quick-cooking oatmeal (uncooked)	1000 mL
½ c.	semi-sweet chocolate chips	125 mL
½ c.	peanut butter	125 mL

Combine margarine, fructose, and water in a small saucepan. Heat until margarine is melted and fructose is completely dissolved. Place the oatmeal in a large mixing bowl. With beater on slow speed, pour margarine mixture into oatmeal. Mix until well blended. Pat into a 15 × 10 in.

(39 × 25 cm) cookie or jelly-roll pan lightly sprayed with oil. Bake at 375 °F (190 °C) for 10 to 15 minutes. Score into 1 × 2 in. (2.5 × 5 cm) bars while warm. Cool completely. Next, melt chocolate chips and peanut butter in a small saucepan. When warm and melted, spread over entire surface of cookie. (I use a pastry brush to do this.) Allow to completely cool. Then cut at scored edges. Remove from pan and store in refrigerator or freezer. My son Bert especially likes this recipe.

Yield: 70 cookies
Exchange, 1 cookie: ⅔ starch/bread
Calories, 1 cookie: 55
Carbohydrates, 1 cookie: 8

Raisin Bars

¾ c.	low-calorie margarine	190 mL
½ c.	granulated fructose	125 mL
2 T.	granulated sugar replacement	30 mL
2	eggs	2
2½ c.	all-purpose flour	625 mL
1 t.	baking soda	5 mL
1 t.	cream of tartar	5 mL
¼ t.	cinnamon	1 mL
¼ t.	nutmeg	1 mL
½ c.	chopped raisins	125 mL
½ c.	skim milk	125 mL

Cream margarine, fructose, and sugar replacement together until thoroughly blended. Beat in eggs, one at a time. Sift together flour, baking soda, cream of tartar, cinnamon, and nutmeg. Fold raisins into flour mixture until well mixed. Add flour mixture alternately with milk to creamed mixture. Then spread in the bottom of a 9×13 in. (23×33 cm) greased baking pan. Bake at 375 °F (190 °C) for 12 to 15 minutes or until done. Allow to cool. Cut into 48 bars.

Yield: 48 cookies
Exchange, 1 cookie: ⅔ starch/bread
Calories, 1 cookie: 53
Carbohydrates, 1 cookie: 8

Date Roll-Ups

1 c.	water	250 mL
½ c.	chopped dates	125 mL
½ c.	low-calorie margarine	125 mL
½ c.	granulated fructose	125 mL
1 T.	hot water	15 mL
1	egg	1
1 t.	vanilla extract	5 mL
2 c.	all-purpose flour	500 mL
½ t.	salt	2 mL
½ t.	baking soda	2 mL

Combine water and dates in a saucepan. While stirring, cook until mixture becomes a purée. (You might want to grind the dates in a blender after they become soft, and then continue cooking.) After mixture becomes thick, allow to cool completely. Then cream together margarine, fructose, and hot water. Add egg and vanilla. Beat until smooth. Sift flour, salt, and baking soda together. Gradually add flour mixture to creamed mixture. Beat until well blended. Divide into three parts and then roll out to ¼-in. (8-mm) thickness. Spread each part with one-third of the date mixture, leaving about ¼ in. (8-mm) around the edges. Roll up jelly-roll fashion. Wrap in plastic wrap and refrigerate to thoroughly chill (at least 3 hours). Slice into ¼-in. (8-mm) cookies. Then bake at 375 °F (190 °C) until brown.

Yield: 66 cookies
Exchange, 1 cookie: ⅓ starch/bread
Calories, 1 cookie: 30
Carbohydrates, 1 cookie: 6

Sour-Cream Cookies

½ c.	low-calorie margarine	125 mL
½ c.	granulated fructose	125 mL
1	egg	1
¼ t.	baking soda	1 mL
¼ c.	dairy, or regular, sour cream	60 mL
½ t.	grated lemon zest	2 mL
½ t.	vanilla extract	2 mL
3 c.	sifted cake flour	750 mL

Cream margarine and fructose together until well blended. Beat in egg.

Dissolve baking soda in sour cream; then beat into creamed mixture. Stir in lemon zest and vanilla. Next, stir in sifted cake flour. (Dough must be firm.) Cut into 50 thin slices. Bake at 375 °F (190 °C) for 8 to 10 minutes, watching cookies carefully to prevent burning.

Yield: 50 cookies
Exchange, 1 cookie: ⅔ starch/bread
Calories, 1 cookie: 50
Carbohydrates, 1 cookie: 7

Ice Cream

Orange Frost

2 c.	skim milk	500 mL
½ c.	low-calorie plain yogurt	125 mL
¼ c.	orange juice	60 mL
2 T.	grated orange rind	30 mL
3 env.	aspartame low-calorie sweetener	3 env.

Combine all ingredients in a bowl. With a rotary beater or electric mixer, beat to blend thoroughly. Pour into ice-cream maker. Freeze to desired consistency, following manufacturer's directions.

Yield: 4 servings
Exchange, 1 serving: 1 skim milk
Calories, 1 serving: 87
Carbohydrates, 1 serving: 12

Pina-Colada Cooler

2 c.	unsweetened pineapple juice	500 mL
¼ c.	unsweetened flaked coconut	60 mL
¼ c.	cold water	60 mL
2 t.	rum flavoring	10 mL

Combine all ingredients in a bowl. Stir to mix. Pour into ice-cream maker. Freeze to desired consistency, following manufacturer's directions.

Yield: 4 servings
Exchange, 1 serving: 1 fruit, ½ fat
Calories, 1 serving: 87
Carbohydrates, 1 serving: 16

Chocolate-Coffee Cream

2 c.	skim milk	500 mL
2 T.	low-calorie instant chocolate-drink mix	30 mL
2 t.	instant coffee, powder	10 mL

Heat milk in the top of a double boiler. Add chocolate-drink mix and instant coffee. Stir to completely dissolve. Cool thoroughly. Pour into ice-cream maker. Freeze to desired consistency, following manufacturer's directions.

Yield: 4 servings
Exchange, 1 serving: ⅔ skim milk
Calories, 1 serving: 60
Carbohydrates, 1 serving: 8

Cooling Stinger

3 c.	skim milk	750 mL
2 T.	brandy flavoring	30 mL
1 T.	wintergreen flavoring	15 mL

Combine all ingredients in a bowl. Stir to mix. Pour into ice-cream maker. Freeze to desired consistency, following manufacturer's directions.

Yield: 4 servings
Exchange, 1 serving: ¾ skim milk
Calories, 1 serving: 68
Carbohydrates, 1 serving: 9

Pink-Petunia Cream

1 qt.	2% low-fat milk	1 L
1 env.	nondairy whipped-topping mix	1 env.
1 T.	cherry flavoring	15 mL
1	egg white, stiffly beaten	1

Combine milk, whipped-topping mix, and cherry flavoring in a bowl. Stir to blend thoroughly. Fold in stiffly beaten egg white. Pour into ice-cream maker, and freeze according to manufacturer's directions.

Yield: 8 servings
Exchange, 1 serving: ¾ low-fat milk
Calories, 1 serving: 92
Carbohydrates, 1 serving: 10

Long-Island Freeze

1 qt.	buttermilk	1 L
3 T.	brandy flavoring	45 mL
3 T.	low-calorie instant chocolate-drink mix	45 mL
1 t.	vanilla extract	5 mL
⅓ c.	mini-chocolate chips	90 mL

Combine buttermilk, brandy flavoring, chocolate-drink mix, and vanilla in a bowl. Stir to mix. Pour into ice-cream maker, and freeze according to manufacturer's directions. Halfway through freezing, add chocolate chips.

Yield: 8 servings
Exchange, 1 serving: ½ starch/bread, ½ skim milk
Calories, 1 serving: 101
Carbohydrates, 1 serving: 13

Apricot-Brandy Freeze

1 qt.	2% low-fat milk	1 L
2 jars (4½ oz. each)	puréed baby peaches	2 jars (126 g each)
2 env.	aspartame low-calorie sweetener	2 env.
2 t.	brandy flavoring	10 mL

Combine all ingredients in a bowl. Stir to blend. Pour into ice-cream maker, and freeze according to manufacturer's directions.

Yield: 8 servings
Exchange, 1 serving: ½ low-fat milk, ½ fruit
Calories, 1 serving: 86
Carbohydrates, 1 serving: 12

Angel-Tip Cooler

2 c.	skim milk	500 mL
1 T.	clear vanilla flavoring	30 mL
1 t.	cornstarch	5 mL

Combine all ingredients in the top of a double boiler. While stirring, cook over simmering water until mixture is slightly thickened. Cool completely. With a rotary beater or electric mixer, beat until slightly fluffy. Turn into ice-cream maker, and freeze according to manufacturer's directions.

Yield: 4 servings
Exchange, 1 serving: ½ skim milk
Calories, 1 serving: 53
Carbohydrates, 1 serving: 6

Cuba Ice

12-oz. can	diet cola	348-g can
2 c.	skim milk	500 mL
2 T.	lime juice	30 mL
1 T.	rum flavoring	15 mL

Combine all ingredients in a bowl. Stir to mix. Pour into ice-cream maker. Freeze to desired consistency, following manufacturer's directions.

Yield: 6 servings
Exchange, 1 serving: ⅓ skim milk
Calories, 1 serving: 31
Carbohydrates, 1 serving: 4

Wild-Irish Freeze

1 qt.	skim milk	1 L
2 T.	nondairy whipped-topping mix	30 mL
3 T.	low-calorie instant chocolate-drink mix	45 mL
1 T.	almond extract	15 mL

Combine all ingredients in a bowl. Stir to completely dissolve chocolate-drink mix. Pour into ice-cream maker, and freeze according to manufacturer's directions.

Yield: 8 servings
Exchange, 1 serving: ½ low-fat milk
Calories, 1 serving: 63
Carbohydrates, 1 serving: 7

Other Desserts

Spicy Orange Slices

2 large	oranges	2 large	
2 T.	all-purpose flour	30 mL	
½ c.	graham-cracker crumbs	125 mL	
½ t.	allspice	2 mL	
	vegetable spray		

Cut oranges (with peel on) into slices about ¼ in. (8 mm) thick, removing the seeds. Combine flour, graham-cracker crumbs, and allspice in a bowl. Stir to mix. Dip orange slices into mixture, making sure to coat well. Place oranges coated with mixture into skillet oiled with vegetable spray. Do not crowd pan. Brown orange slices on both sides. Respray pan if necessary.

Yield: 8 servings
Exchange, 1 serving: ½ starch/bread
Calories, 1 serving: 40
Carbohydrates, 1 serving: 7

Almond Bavarian

2 env.	unflavored gelatin	2 env.	
1½ c.	skim milk	375 mL	
¾ c.	chopped blanched almonds	190 mL	
¼ c.	granulated fructose	60 mL	
6	egg yolks, slightly beaten	6	
1 t.	vanilla extract	5 mL	
¾ t.	almond extract	4 mL	
1 qt.	prepared nondairy whipped topping	1 L	

Soften gelatin in ½ c. (125 mL) of the skim milk. Combine remaining skim milk, almonds, fructose, and egg yolks in the top of a double boiler. Cook and stir over simmering water until smooth and thickened. Remove from heat. Stir in extracts and softened gelatin. Continue stirring to completely dissolve gelatin. Chill mixture until the consistency of egg whites. Fold in nondairy whipped topping. Transfer to a lightly greased 2-qt. (2-L) salad mould. Chill until firm.

Yield: 16 servings
Exchange, 1 serving: ½ low-fat milk, ½ fat
Calories, 1 serving: 85
Carbohydrates, 1 serving: 10

Orange Ambrosia

2	tangerines	2
1	orange	1
⅓ c.	pineapple cubes	90 mL
1 T.	granulated fructose	15 mL
1 T.	unsweetened shredded coconut	15 mL

With a sharp knife, section tangerines and orange. Remove membranes and seeds. Arrange fruit sections and pineapple cubes in layers in three dessert glasses, sprinkling each layer with small amount of fructose. Top each dessert glass with one-third of the shredded coconut. Chill thoroughly before serving.

Yield: 3 servings
Exchange, 1 serving: 1 fruit
Calories, 1 serving: 76
Carbohydrates, 1 serving: 14

Gingered Cantaloupe

1	cantaloupe	1
½ t.	ginger	2 mL
2 t.	honey	10 mL

Cut cantaloupe in half; then remove seeds and rind. Cut into very thin slices. Arrange slices in a fan on a large plate. Sprinkle with ginger. Warm the honey and then drizzle it over top of cantaloupe slices.

Yield: 4 servings
Exchange, 1 serving: ¾ fruit
Calories, 1 serving: 45
Carbohydrates, 1 serving: 9

Hazelnut Delight

2	eggs	2
½ c.	granulated sugar replacement	125 mL
2 T.	all-purpose flour	30 mL
½ t.	baking powder	2 mL
dash	salt	dash
½ c.	finely chopped apples	125 mL
⅓ c.	finely chopped hazelnuts	90 mL

Beat eggs and sugar replacement together until foamy. Beat in flour, baking powder, and salt. Next, stir in apples and hazelnuts. Transfer to greased 8-in. (20-cm) pie pan. Bake at 325 °F (165 °C) for 25 to 30 minutes or until set. Chill and then cut into wedges.

Yield: 8 servings
Exchange, 1 serving: 1 fruit
Calories, 1 serving: 72
Carbohydrates, 1 serving: 13

Fruit Bowl

1 c.	water	250 mL
1 env.	unflavored gelatin	1 env.
6-oz. can	frozen tangerine juice	180-g can
2	grapefruits	2
4	oranges	4
1	avocado	1

Sprinkle gelatin over water in a small saucepan. Allow to soften for 5 minutes. Bring to a boil, stirring to dissolve gelatin. Remove from heat; then stir in frozen tangerine juice. Allow to cool but not thicken. Peel and section grapefruits and oranges, removing seeds and membranes. Peel, pit, and thinly slice avocado. Arrange fruit as desired in six dessert dishes. Pour tangerine gelatin over fruit to fill dishes. Chill thoroughly.

Yield: 8 servings
Exchange, 1 serving: 2 fruit, 1 fat
Calories, 1 serving: 155
Carbohydrates, 1 serving: 28

Rhubarb with Cheese

1 qt.	rhubarb	1 L
½ c.	granulated fructose	125 mL
½ c.	soft white-bread crumbs	125 mL
⅓ c.	grated Cheddar cheese	90 mL

Place half of the rhubarb in a layer on the bottom of a lightly greased baking dish. Sprinkle with half of the fructose. Place half of the bread crumbs in a layer on top. Repeat layers. Sprinkle the cheese over the top. Bake at 350 °F (175 °C) for 30 to 35 minutes or until rhubarb is tender and cheese is browned.

Yield: 8 servings
Exchange, 1 serving: ½ starch/bread, 1 fat
Calories, 1 serving: 91
Carbohydrates, 1 serving: 8

Persimmon Mould

⅓ c.	low-calorie margarine	90 mL
1 c.	granulated brown-sugar replacement	250 mL
3	eggs	3
1½ c.	sifted all-purpose flour	375 mL
2 t.	baking powder	10 mL
½ c.	skim milk	125 mL
1½ c.	persimmon pulp	375 mL
½ t. each	cinnamon, nutmeg	2 mL each

Beat margarine and brown-sugar replacement together until light and fluffy. Add eggs, one at a time, beating well after each addition. Combine flour and baking powder in a bowl. Add flour mixture to eggs alternately with milk, beginning and ending with flour. Fold in persimmon pulp, cinnamon, and nutmeg. Transfer to a 1½-qt. (1½-L) lightly greased baking dish. Place baking dish in a pan of water. (Water should reach halfway up sides of baking dish. Add extra water if needed while baking.) Bake at 325 °F (165 °C) for 50 to 60 minutes or until custard tests done.

Yield: 10 servings
Exchange, 1 serving: 1 fruit, 1 starch/bread
Calories, 1 serving: 136
Carbohydrates, 1 serving: 30

Fried Apples

6 large	tart apples	6 large
½ c.	all-purpose flour	125 mL
2 T.	granulated fructose	30 mL
1 t.	nutmeg	5 mL
dash	cloves	dash
	vegetable spray	

Core apples and then cut them into ½-in. (1.25-cm) slices (do not peel). Combine flour, fructose, nutmeg, and cloves in a bowl. Stir to blend. Lightly coat each side of the apples slices with the flour mixture. Fry in a vegetable-sprayed skillet until golden brown on both sides. Respray pan as needed.

Yield: 12 servings
Exchange, 1 serving: 1 fruit, ¼ starch/bread
Calories, 1 serving: 78
Carbohydrates, 1 serving: 16

Apple-Cider Raisin Delight

1½ c.	water	375 mL
1½ c.	apple cider	375 mL
1 c.	raisins	250 mL
1 c.	chopped apples	250 mL
3 T.	lemon juice	45 mL
1 T.	low-calorie margarine	15 mL
1 t.	cinnamon	5 mL
½ t.	salt	2 mL
3 T.	cornstarch	45 mL

Reserve ½ c. (125 mL) of the water. Combine the remaining 1 c. (250 mL) of water with the apple cider, raisins, apples, lemon juice, margarine, cinnamon, and salt in a saucepan. Bring to a boil. Now combine the reserved ½ c. (125 mL) of water with the cornstarch. Pour into the apple mixture. Cook and stir until thick. Cool slightly. Transfer to a serving dish. Cool completely.

Yield: 12 servings
Exchange, 1 serving: 1¼ fruit
Calories, 1 serving: 72
Carbohydrates, 1 serving: 18

Fried Bananas

6	bananas	6
dash	salt and pepper	dash
1 T.	fresh lemon juice	15 mL
1	egg	1
2 t.	water	10 mL
½ c.	dry bread crumbs	125 mL

Peel and cut bananas in half crosswise and then lengthwise. (Each banana should yield four pieces.) Sprinkle the banana wedges with salt, pepper, and lemon juice. Combine egg and water in a flat-bottomed bowl. Beat with fork to completely blend. Dip and roll banana in the egg mixture. Roll in the bread crumbs. Shake off any excess crumbs. Fry in deep fat at 325 °F (165 °C) until golden brown.

Yield: 24 servings
Exchange, 1 serving: ½ fruit
Calories, 1 serving: 25
Carbohydrates, 1 serving: 7

✳ Graham-Cracker Cherry Dessert *Pineapple*

15	graham crackers	15
5-oz. can	crushed pineapple, in its own juice	149-g can
2 t.	cornstarch	10 mL
½ c.	chopped walnuts	125 mL
2 pkgs.*	sugar-free cherry gelatin	2 pkgs.*

*four-servings size

Crush graham crackers into fine crumbs. Line the bottom of an 8-in. (20-cm)-square baking pan with half of the crumbs. Refrigerate. In a saucepan, combine crushed pineapple, in its own juice, and the cornstarch. Stir to blend. Cook over low heat until mixture thickens. Cool completely. Fold in walnuts. Now spread mixture over the top of the crumbs in the pan. Sprinkle with remaining crumbs. Lightly pat down the surface. Refrigerate. Make gelatin as directed on package. Allow gelatin to set to the consistency of egg whites. Pour over the top layer of crumbs. Refrigerate until firm.

Yield: 8 servings
Exchange, 1 serving: ⅔ starch/bread, 1 fat
Calories, 1 serving: 105
Carbohydrates, 1 serving: 12

Strawberry Dream

1 qt.	strawberries	1 L
¼ c.	granulated fructose	60 mL
½ c.	quick-cooking tapioca	125 mL
¼ t.	salt	1 mL
2 c.	boiling water	500 mL
2 c.	prepared nondairy whipped topping	500 mL

Reserve five strawberries for garnish. Crush remaining strawberries and mix them with fructose. Allow to stand at least an hour. Mix tapioca with salt and boiling water. Cook over low heat, stirring constantly, until tapioca is clear. Drain juice from berries into a measuring cup. Add enough water to berry juice to make 2 cups (500 mL) of liquid. Stir in crushed strawberries. Stir into tapioca mixture and cook 6 minutes longer. Cool completely. Divide half of the tapioca mixture among 10 dessert dishes. Fold the nondairy whipped topping into the remaining tapioca mixture; then divide it evenly among the dessert dishes. Now cut the reserved strawberries in half, and use them to garnish the top of each dish. Chill thoroughly before serving.

Yield: 10 servings
Exchange, 1 serving: ½ starch/bread, ½ fruit
Calories, 1 serving: 72
Carbohydrates, 1 serving: 14

Peach Slump

6 c.	sliced peaches (peeled)	1500 mL
⅓ c.	granulated fructose	90 mL
1½ t.	cinnamon	7 mL
½ c.	water	125 mL
12	unbaked biscuits	12
12 T.	prepared nondairy whipped topping	180 mL

Combine peaches, fructose, cinnamon, and water in a nonstick skillet. Bring to a simmer. Top with biscuits. Cover and simmer for 25 to 30 minutes. Top each serving with 1 T. (15 mL) of nondairy whipped topping.

Yield: 12 servings
Exchange, 1 serving: 1 starch/bread, 1 fruit
Calories, 1 serving: 112
Carbohydrates, 1 serving: 19

Brandied Apples

6	tart apples	6
1 T.	lemon juice	15 mL
¼ c.	brandy	60 mL
⅛ t.	cinnamon	½ mL
12 T.	prepared nondairy whipped topping	180 mL

Core apples and then cut them into quarters. Place quarters in a bowl. Sprinkle with lemon juice, tossing to coat. Drain off any excess lemon juice. Pour brandy and cinnamon over apple quarters, tossing to coat. Cover tightly and marinate for several hours or overnight. Toss several times during marinating. For each of the 12 servings, place two quarters in a small dessert dish and top with 1 T. (15 mL) nondairy whipped topping.

Yield: 12 servings
Exchange, 1 serving: 1 fruit
Calories, 1 serving: 57
Carbohydrates, 1 serving: 13

Lemon Meringue Nests

2	egg whites	2
1 t.	sorbitol	5 mL
1 t.	white vinegar	5 mL
1 t.	clear vanilla flavoring	5 mL
1 pkg.*	sugar-free lemon instant pudding and pie filling	1 pkg.*
1½ c.	cold skim milk	375 mL

*four-servings size

Beat egg whites until stiff. Gradually beat in sorbitol, vinegar, and vanilla. Continue beating until very stiff. Shape egg-white mixture into four nestlike forms on a lightly greased cookie sheet. Bake at 250 °F (125 °C) for 35 to 40 minutes or until surface becomes crusty. Allow to cool in oven or move to cooling rack. Combine pudding mix and skim milk in a bowl. Whip to blend. Refrigerate until completely set. Then spoon into meringue nests. Store in refrigerator.

Yield: 4 servings
Exchange, 1 serving: 1 starch/bread
Calories, 1 serving: 77
Carbohydrates, 1 serving: 16

Hidden Apple ✓

1	cored apple	1
2 T.	orange juice	30 mL
dash each	nutmeg, cinnamon, sugar replacement	dash each
	uncooked dough for 1 biscuit	

Prick the inside of the apple cavity with a fork or toothpick. Sprinkle with orange juice, spices, and sugar replacement. Place the biscuit dough on a lightly floured surface. Flatten the dough into a square that is large enough to wrap completely around the apple. Place the apple in the middle of the dough. Bring the corners of the dough up to the top of the apple. Secure with a toothpick or press the edges together firmly. Place in a baking dish. Then bake at 375 °F (190 °C) for 20 to 25 minutes or until done.

Yield: 1 serving
Exchange, 1 serving: 1 fruit, 1 starch/bread
Calories, 1 serving: 135
Carbohydrates, 1 serving: 29

Date Nut Dish ✓

2	eggs	2
1 T.	granulated sugar replacement	15 mL
⅔ c.	all-purpose flour	180 mL
1 t.	baking powder	5 mL
½ c.	coarsely chopped walnuts	125 mL
1 c.	chopped dates	250 mL

Beat eggs until thick and lemon colored. Stir in sugar replacement. Combine flour and baking powder in sifter; then sift into egg mixture. Beat until well blended. Fold in walnuts and dates. Transfer to a well greased 9-in. (23-cm) layer cake pan. Bake at 350 °F (175 °C) for 20 to 30 minutes or until golden brown on top. Serve warm.

Yield: 10 servings
Exchange, 1 serving: 1 fruit, ½ starch/bread, ½ fat
Calories, 1 serving: 131
Carbohydrates, 1 serving: 22

Crusts

Cocoa-Flavored Crisp-Cereal Crust

| 2 c. | cocoa-flavored cereal | 500 mL |
| 1½ T. | water | 21 mL |

In a food processor, blend the dry cereal on HIGH until it becomes a medium-fine grain. Add water and then process for another minute. Press mixture into an ungreased 8- or 9-in. (20- or 23-cm) pie pan.

Yield: 8 servings or single pie crust
Exchange, 1 serving: ⅓ starch/bread
Calories, 1 serving: 25
Carbohydrates, 1 serving: 4

Graham-Cracker Crust

20	2-in. (5-cm)-square graham crackers	20
2 T.	water	30 mL
½ t.	cinnamon	2 mL

Using food processor, crush crackers to make a cup of fine crumbs. Add water and cinnamon. Blend until sticky. Press mixture into an ungreased 8- or 9-in. (20- or 23-cm) pie pan.

Yield: 8 servings or single pie crust
Exchange, 1 serving: ¾ starch/bread
Calories, 1 serving: 68
Carbohydrates, 1 serving: 12

Cocoa-Flavored Puffed-Cereal Crust

| 2½ c. | cocoa-flavored cereal | 625 mL |
| 1½ T. | water | 21 mL |

Blend dry cereal on HIGH in a food processor. Add water and then blend for another minute. Press mixture into ungreased 8- or 9-in. (20- or 23-cm) pie pan.

Yield: 8 servings or single pie crust
Exchange, 1 serving: ⅓ starch/bread
Calories, 1 serving: 27
Carbohydrates, 1 serving: 5

Ginger-Cookie Crust #1

| 20 | 2-in. (5-cm) ginger cookies | 20 |
| 1 T. | water | 15 mL |

Blend cookies on HIGH in a food processor. Add water and blend until moist. Press crust into ungreased 8- or 9-in. (20- or 23-cm) pan.

Yield: 8 servings or single pie crust
Exchange, 1 serving: ¾ starch/bread
Calories, 1 serving: 56
Carbohydrates, 1 serving: 13

Ginger-Cookie Crust #2

| 20 | 2-in. (5-cm) ginger cookies | 20 |
| 2 T. | skim milk | 30 mL |

Crush cookies in food processor on HIGH. Process until crumbs become very fine. Add milk and process until dough forms a ball. Press into ungreased 8- or 9-in. (20- or 23-cm) pie pan or torte pan, or chill and roll dough.

Yield: 8 servings or single pie crust
Exchange, 1 serving: ¾ starch/bread
Calories, 1 serving: 56
Carbohydrates, 1 serving: 13

Corn-Cereal Crust

3 c.	cornflake cereal	750 mL
1½ T.	water	21 mL

Crush cornflakes in food processor on HIGH to make 1¼-c. (310-mL) of fine crumbs. Add water and blend until moist. Press crust into ungreased 8- or 9-in. (20- or 23-cm) pie pan.

Yield: 8 servings or single pie crust
Exchange, 1 serving: ½ starch/bread
Calories, 1 serving: 35
Carbohydrates, 1 serving: 8

Bran-Cereal-with-Raisins Crust

2 c.	raisin bran cereal	500 mL
2 t.	rum flavoring	10 mL

Using a blender, chop cereal thoroughly, one cup at a time. Make sure to stir cereal from underneath blender's blades when blender is turned off. Transfer to food processor and add rum flavoring. Process until sticky. Press mixture into ungreased 8- or 9-in. (20- or 23-cm) pie pan.

Yield: 8 servings or single pie crust
Exchange, 1 serving: ½ starch/bread
Calories, 1 serving: 35
Carbohydrates, 1 serving: 8

Cinnamon-Crunch Cereal Crust

3 c.	cinnamon cereal	750 mL
1½ T.	water	21 mL

Crush cereal on HIGH in food processor until crumbs become fine. Add water and blend to moisten. Press crumbs into ungreased 8- or 9-in. (20-or 23-cm) pie pan.

Yield: 8 servings or single pie crust
Exchange, 1 serving: ⅔ starch/bread
Calories, 1 serving: 50
Carbohydrates, 1 serving: 12

Meringue Crust

3	egg whites, at room temperature	3
¼ t.	cream of tartar	1 mL
dash	salt	dash
¼ c.	granulated sugar replacement	60 mL

Combine egg whites, cream of tartar, and salt in a mixing bowl. Beat until soft peaks form. Gradually add sugar replacement. Beat to stiff peaks. Spread over bottom and sides of 8- or 9-in. (20- or 23-cm) pie pan. Bake at 275 °F (135 °C) for an hour or until lightly browned and crisp. Cool before filling.

Yield: 8 servings
Exchange, 1 serving: negligible
Calories, 1 serving: negligible
Carbohydrates, 1 serving: negligible

Flavored-Meringue Crust

3	egg whites, at room temperature	3
¼ t.	cream of tartar	1 mL
dash	salt	dash
1 t.	one of the following:	5 mL
	any type of flavoring	
	vanilla extract	
	ground cardamom	
	nutmeg	
	cinnamon	
	lavender leaves	
	pumpkin-pie spice	
	mace	
	lemon juice	

Combine egg whites, cream of tartar, and salt in a mixing bowl. Beat until soft peaks form. Add flavoring of your choice. Beat to stiff peaks. Spread over bottom and sides of 8- or 9-in. (20- or 23-cm) pie pan. Bake at 275 °F (135 °C) for an hour or until lightly browned and crisp. Cool before filling.

Yield: 8 servings
Exchange, 1 serving: negligible
Calories, 1 serving: negligible
Carbohydrates, 1 serving: negligible

Orange Crust

3 c.	all-purpose flour	750 mL
1 c.	solid shortening	250 mL
1 t.	granulated sugar replacement	5 mL
2 t.	grated orange peel	10 mL
7 T.	orange juice	105 mL

Combine flour, shortening, sugar replacement, and orange peel in a bowl or food processor. Cut until mixture is the consistency of cornmeal. Make a well in the middle of the mixture; then add orange juice. Toss until mixture is moist enough to hold a shape. If needed, add a small amount of water, 1 t. (5 mL) at a time. Form into a ball, wrap in plastic wrap, and chill for at least 2 hours. Then divide dough in half. Roll out both halves on a lightly floured surface. Arrange bottom crust in pie pan. Add filling. Adjust top crust, scoring or cutting slits to allow steam to escape. Seal edges. Bake as directed in your pie recipe.

Yield: 8 servings or double pie crust
Exchange, 1 serving: 2 starch/bread, 3 fat
Calories, 1 serving: 310
Carbohydrates, 1 serving: 30

Puff Paste

1 c.	unsalted butter	250 mL
2 c.	sifted cake flour	500 mL
½ c.	ice water	125 mL

Cut ⅓ c. (90 mL) of butter into the cake flour. Allow the remaining butter to become soft but not runny. Add ice water to flour mixture, 1 T. (15 mL) at a time, until a soft dough forms. Chill for an hour. Then roll out dough on a lightly floured surface. Brush with one-fourth of the softened butter. Fold in half, brush with 2 T. (30 mL) of the softened butter, and fold in half again. Place in plastic wrap and chill for an hour. Then roll out and repeat brushing with half of the remaining softened butter. Repeat process a third time with the remaining butter. This can be baked immediately as directed in your pie recipe, refrigerated for up to 2 days, or frozen.

Yield: 16 servings
Exchange, 1 serving: 1 starch/bread, 2½ fat
Calories, 1 serving: 140
Carbohydrates, 1 serving: 16

Cottage-Cheese Crust

⅓ c.	butter-flavored shortening	90 mL
1 c.	sifted all-purpose flour	250 mL
½ c.	low-calorie cottage cheese	125 mL

Cut shortening into flour; then add cottage cheese and mix into a smooth dough. Wrap dough in plastic wrap and chill for at least an hour. Roll to desired shape.

Yield: 8 servings or single pie crust
Exchange, 1 serving: ⅔ starch/bread, 1½ fat
Calories, 1 serving: 156
Carbohydrates, 1 serving: 12

Cheddar-Cheese Crust

1½ c.	all-purpose flour	375 mL
dash	salt	dash
¾ c.	grated sharp Cheddar cheese	190 mL
½ c.	solid shortening	125 mL
5 to 6 T.	ice water	75 to 90 mL

Combine flour, salt, cheese, and shortening in a food processor with a steel blade. Process on HIGH with alternate on/off switch until mixture turns into coarse crumbs. On LOW, add water through the feeder tube, 1 T. (15 mL) at a time, until dough starts to ball. Form dough into a ball with your hands. Wrap in plastic wrap and chill for 2 hours. Then divide dough in half and roll out both halves on lightly floured surface. Arrange bottom crust in pie pan. Add filling. Adjust top crust, scoring or cutting slits to allow steam to escape. Seal edges. Bake as directed in your pie recipe.

Yield: 8 servings or double pie crust
Exchange, 1 serving: 1 starch/bread, 2½ fat
Calories, 1 serving: 200
Carbohydrates, 1 serving: 15

Egg-Yolk Crust

1 c.	sifted all-purpose flour	250 mL
dash	salt	dash
1 T.	granulated sugar replacement	15 mL
¼ c.	butter-flavored shortening	60 mL
1	egg yolk, slightly beaten	1

Combine flour, salt, and sugar replacement in food processor or bowl. Cut in shortening, using on/off switch or short cuts. Add egg yolk and mix thoroughly. Press dough into bottom of 8- or 9-in. (20- or 23-cm) pie pan, springform pan, or tart pans. Add filling as directed in your pie recipe or fill with pie weights. Bake at 425 °F (220 °C) for 10 minutes or until crust is slightly brown.

Yield: 8 servings or single pie crust
Exchange, 1 serving: ⅔ starch/bread, 1 fat
Calories, 1 serving: 115
Carbohydrates, 1 serving: 12

Pastry Crust

2 c.	sifted all-purpose flour	500 mL
dash	salt	dash
1 c.	butter-flavored shortening	250 mL
⅓ c.	ice water	90 mL

Combine flour and salt in bowl or food processor. Cut in shortening until mixture is in fine crumbs. Add water and mix to a dough. Chill for an hour. Divide dough in half. Roll out half on lightly floured surface. Line pan, fill, and then roll out top crust. Slit top crust to allow steam to escape. Place on top of filling and seal edges. Bake as directed in your pie recipe.

Yield: 8 servings or double pie crust
Exchange, 1 serving: 1⅓ starch/bread, 5 fat
Calories, 1 serving: 326
Carbohydrates, 1 serving: 21

Toppings

Pecan Topping

½ c.	granulated brown-sugar replacement	125 mL
½ c.	finely chopped pecans	125 mL
¼ c.	all-purpose flour	60 mL
¼ c.	low-calorie margarine	60 mL

Combine all ingredients. Toss and stir with a fork until completely mixed.

Yield: 8 servings
Exchange, 1 serving: 1⅔ fat
Calories, 1 serving: 75
Carbohydrates, 1 serving: 3

Caramelized-Pecan Topping

⅔ c.	coarsely chopped pecans	180 mL
2 T.	low-calorie margarine	30 mL
⅓ c.	granulated fructose	90 mL

Place pecans in small skillet over medium heat and toast slightly. Add margarine and allow to melt. Stir in fructose. Allow to cool. Stir until mixture becomes thick. Pour out onto waxed paper and allow to cool.

Yield: 8 servings
Exchange, 1 serving: ½ fruit, 1½ fat
Calories, 1 serving: 97
Carbohydrates, 1 serving: 7

Coconut Topping

2	egg whites, slightly beaten	2
2 T.	granulated sugar replacement	30 mL
⅓ c.	unsweetened grated coconut	90 mL

Combine egg whites and sugar replacement in a medium-size mixing bowl. Beat until soft peaks form. Fold in coconut. Spoon topping onto top of cool pie filling. Spread gently with the back of the spoon. Broil on bottom rack of oven for 5 to 6 minutes. Watch carefully because this topping tends to burn.

Yield: 8 servings
Exchange, 1 serving: negligible
Calories, 1 serving: 11
Carbohydrates, 1 serving: negligible

Ginger-Crumb Topping

12	gingersnaps	12
2 T.	all-purpose flour	30 mL
1 T.	hot water	15 mL

Break gingersnaps and place in blender. Blend into fine crumbs. Combine gingersnap crumbs and flour in a bowl. Stir to mix. Add hot water and stir until mixture turns to crumbs.

Yield: 8 servings
Exchange, 1 serving: ½ starch/bread
Calories, 1 serving: 40
Carbohydrates, 1 serving: 11

Brazil-Nut Topping

⅔ c.	coarsely chopped Brazil nuts	180 mL
1 T.	granulated fructose	15 mL
⅓ c.	graham-cracker crumbs	90 mL

Toast Brazil nuts in a small skillet over low heat until lightly browned. Sprinkle with fructose. Shake pan to coat nuts. Stir in graham-cracker crumbs. Remove from heat and allow to cool.

Yield: 8 servings
Exchange, 1 serving: ⅓ starch/bread, ⅓ fat
Calories, 1 serving: 102
Carbohydrates, 1 serving: 5

Estee's Fudgy Fructose Frosting

1 c.	fructose	250 mL
⅔ c.	skim milk	180 mL
2 T.	cornstarch	30 mL
2 sq. (1 oz. each)	unsweetened chocolate	2 sq. (30 g each)
2 T.	margarine (corn oil)	30 mL
1 t.	vanilla extract	5 mL

Mix fructose, skim milk, and cornstarch together in saucepan until cornstarch dissolves. Add chocolate and cook over medium heat until chocolate melts and mixture thickens and bubbles. Remove from heat. Add margarine and vanilla, stirring until creamy. Spread over cake.

Yield: 20 servings
Exchange, 1 serving: 1 fruit, ½ fat
Calories, 1 serving: 70
Carbohydrates, 1 serving: 12

Estee's Cream-Cheese Frosting ⌐

8 oz.	cream cheese	240 g
¼ c.	margarine (corn oil)	60 mL
½ c.	fructose	125 mL
½ t.	vanilla extract (optional)	2 mL

Beat cream cheese, margarine and fructose together in mixer until smooth. Add vanilla, if desired, and continue beating until creamy. Spread over cake.

Yield: 20 servings
Exchange, 1 serving: ⅓ fruit, 1 fat
Calories, 1 serving: 80
Carbohydrates, 1 serving: 5

Lemon-Crumb Topping ⌐

½ c.	all-purpose flour	125 mL
¼ c.	granulated sugar replacement	60 mL
2 t.	grated lemon peel	10 mL
¼ c.	cold low-calorie margarine	60 mL

Combine flour, sugar replacement, and lemon peel in a mixing bowl.

Toss to mix. Cut cold margarine into lemon mixture until mixture turns to crumbs.

Yield: 8 servings
Exchange, 1 serving: negligible
Calories, 1 serving: 26
Carbohydrates, 1 serving: 5

Oatmeal-Crumb Topping

½ c.	quick-cooking oatmeal (uncooked)	125 mL
⅓ c.	granulated brown-sugar replacement	90 mL
2 T.	granulated fructose	30 mL
¼ c.	all-purpose flour	60 mL
¼ c.	cold low-calorie margarine	60 mL

Combine oatmeal, brown-sugar replacement, fructose, and flour in a bowl. Stir to mix. Cut cold margarine into mixture until mixture turns to crumbs.

Yield: 8 servings
Exchange, 1 serving: ½ starch/bread, ½ fat
Calories, 1 serving: 70
Carbohydrates, 1 serving: 7

Raisin Topping

3 slices	white bread	3 slices
⅓ c.	raisins	90 mL
2 t.	all-purpose flour	10 mL
1 T.	granulated fructose	15 mL

Cut crusts from bread and allow bread to dry completely. Break bread into pieces and place in a blender. Blend into coarse crumbs. Toss raisins in flour. Add to bread crumbs in blender. Blend until mixed and raisins are slightly chopped. Then blend in fructose.

Yield: 8 servings
Exchange, 1 serving: ¼ starch/bread, ½ fruit
Calories, 1 serving: 51
Carbohydrates, 1 serving: 12

Two Egg-Whites Meringue

2	egg whites, at room temperature	2
¼ t.	cream of tartar	1 mL
dash	salt	dash
¼ t.	vanilla extract	1 mL
3 T.	granulated sugar replacement	45 mL

Combine egg whites, cream of tartar, and salt in a medium-size mixing bowl. Beat until mixture is frothy. Gradually add vanilla and sugar replacement, ½ T. (7 mL) at a time. Beat until meringue is stiff.

For topping: Bake at 350 °F (175 °C) for 10 to 12 minutes.

For shells: Bake at 250 °F (120 °C) for 40 to 50 minutes. Turn off oven, allowing shells to remain in oven until cool.

Yield: 4 to 8 servings
Exchange: negligible
Calories: negligible
Carbohydrates: negligible

Three Egg-Whites Meringue

3	egg whites, at room temperature	3
¼ t.	cream of tartar	1 mL
¼ t.	salt	1 mL
½ t.	vanilla extract	2 mL
⅔ c.	granulated sugar replacement	180 mL

Combine egg whites, cream of tartar, and salt in a medium-size mixing bowl. Beat until mixture is frothy. Gradually add vanilla and sugar replacement, 1 T. (15 mL) at a time. Beat until meringue is stiff.

Fop topping: Bake at 350 °F (175 °C) for 10 to 12 minutes.

For shells: Bake at 250 °F (120 °C) for 40 to 50 minutes. Turn off oven, allowing shells to remain in oven until cool.

Yield: 6 to 8 servings
Exchange: negligible
Calories: negligible
Carbohydrates: negligible

Meringue with Sorbitol

2	egg whites, at room temperature	2
½ t.	cream of tartar	2 mL
2 t.	sorbitol	10 mL
1 t.	vanilla extract	5 mL

Combine egg whites and cream of tartar in a medium-size mixing bowl. Beat until mixture is frothy. Gradually add sorbitol and vanilla. Beat until meringue is stiff.

For topping: Bake at 350 °F (175 °C) for 10 to 12 minutes.

For shells: Bake at 250 °F (120 °C) for 40 to 50 minutes. Turn off oven, allowing shells to remain in oven until cool.

Yield: 4 to 8 servings
Exchange: negligible
Calories: negligible
Carbohydrates: negligible

Estee's Lemon Chiffon Frosting

1 c.	fructose	250 mL
¼ c.	water	60 mL
2	egg whites	2
½ t.	cream of tartar	2 mL
1½ t.	lemon flavoring	7 mL
2 drops	yellow food coloring	2 drops

Mix fructose and water in saucepan and cook over medium heat until fructose is completely dissolved. Continue cooking and stirring until syrup comes to a boil. Remove from heat. Now beat egg whites and cream of tartar together with electric mixer until soft peaks form. Gradually add fructose syrup in a thin stream while beating (this should take about 5 minutes). Add lemon flavoring and coloring; then beat for about 2 minutes or until stiff and glossy. Spread over cake.

Yield: 20 servings
Exchange, 1 serving: 1 fruit
Calories, 1 serving: 40
Carbohydrates, 1 serving: 10

EXCHANGE LISTS

FOR MEAL PLANNING

The reason for dividing food into six different groups is that foods vary in their carbohydrate, protein, fat, and calorie content. Each exchange list contains foods that are alike – each choice contains about the same amount of carbohydrate, protein, fat, and calories.

The following chart shows the amount of these nutrients in one serving from each exchange list.

Exchange List	Carbohydrate (grams)	Protein (grams)	Fat (grams)	Calories
Starch/Bread	15	3	trace	80
Meat				
Lean	--	7	3	55
Medium-Fat	–	7	5	75
High-Fat	–	7	8	100
Vegetable	5	2	–	25
Fruit	15	–	–	60
Milk				
Skim	12	8	trace	90
Low-fat	12	8	5	120
Whole	12	8	8	150
Fat	–	–	5	45

As you read the exchange lists, you will notice that one choice often is a larger amount of food than another choice from the same list. Because foods are so different, each food is measured or weighed so the amount of carbohydrate, protein, fat, and calories is the same in each choice.

You will notice symbols on some foods in the exchange groups. Foods that are high in fiber (3 grams or more per normal serving) have this ☞ symbol. High fiber foods are good for you. It is important to eat more of these foods.

Foods that are high in sodium (400 milligrams or more of sodium per normal serving) have this ☞ symbol. It's a good idea to limit your intake of high salt foods, especially if you have high blood pressure.

If you have a favorite food that is not included in any of these groups, ask your dietitian about it. That food can probably be worked into your meal plan, at least now and then.

*The exchange lists are the basis of a meal planning system designed by a committee of the American Diabetes Association and the American Dietetic Association. While designed primarily for people with diabetes and others who must follow special diets, the exchange lists are based on principles of good nutrition that apply to everyone. ©1986 American Diabetes Association, American Dietetic Association.

1
Starch/Bread List

Each item in this list contains approximately 15 grams of carbohydrate, 3 grams of protein, a trace of fat, and 80 calories. Whole grain products average about 2 grams o fiber per serving. Some foods are higher in fiber. Those food that contain 3 or more grams of fiber per serving are identifie with the fiber symbol ✍

You can choose your starch exchanges from any of the items on this list. If you want to eat a starch food that is not on this list, the general rule is that:

- 1/2 cup of cereal, grain or pasta is one servi
- 1 ounce of a bread product is one serving.

Your dietitian can help you be more exact.

CEREALS/GRAINS/PASTA

✍ Bran cereals, concentrated	1/3 cup
✍ Bran cereals, flaked	1/2 cup
(such as Bran Buds,® All Bran®)	
Bulgur (cooked)	1/2 cup
Cooked cereals	1/2 cup
Cornmeal (dry)	2 1/2 Tbsp.
Grapenuts	3 Tbsp.
Grits (cooked)	1/2 cup
Other ready-to-eat unsweetened cereals	3/4 cup
Pasta (cooked)	1/2 cup
Puffed cereal	1 1/2 cup
Rice, white or brown (cooked)	1/3 cup
Shredded wheat	1/2 cup
✍ Wheat germ	3 Tbsp.

DRIED BEANS/PEAS/LENTILS

✍ Beans and peas (cooked) (such as kidney, white, split, blackeye)	1/3 cup
✍ Lentils (cooked)	1/3 cup
✍ Baked beans	1/4 cup

STARCHY VEGETABLES

✍ Corn	1/2 cup
✍ Corn on cob, 6 in. long	1
✍ Lima beans	1/2 cup
✍ Peas, green (canned or frozen)	1/2 cup
✍ Plantain	1/2 cup
Potato, baked	1 small (3 oz.)
Potato, mashed	1/2 cup
Squash, winter (acorn, butternut)	3/4 cup
Yam, sweet potato, plain	1/3 cup

BREAD

Bagel	1/2 (1 oz.)
Bread sticks, crisp, 4 in. long x 1/2 in.	2 (2/3 oz.)
Croutons, low fat	1 cup
English muffin	1/2
Frankfurter or hamburger bun	1/2 (1 oz.)
Pita, 6 in. across	1/2
Plain roll, small	1 (1 oz.)
Raisin, unfrosted	1 slice (1 oz.)
✍ Rye, pumpernickel	1 slice (1 oz.)
Tortilla, 6 in. across	1
White (including French, Italian)	1 slice (1 oz.)
Whole wheat	1 slice (1 oz.)

CRACKERS/SNACKS

Animal crackers	8
Graham crackers, 2 1/2 in. square	3
Matzoth	3/4 oz.
Melba toast	5 slices
Oyster crackers	24
Popcorn (popped, no fat added)	3 cups
Pretzels	3/4 oz.
Rye crisp, 2 in. x 3 1/2 in.	4
Saltine-type crackers	6
Whole wheat crackers, no fat added (crisp breads, such as Finn® Kavli®, Wasa®)	2-4 slices (3/4

STARCH FOODS PREPARED WITH FA·

(Count as 1 starch/bread serving, plus 1 fat serving.)

Biscuit, 2 1/2 in. across	1
Chow mein noodles	1/2 cup
Corn bread, 2 in. cube	1 (2 oz.)
Cracker, round butter type	6
French fried potatoes, 2 in. to 3 1/2 in. long	10 (1 1/2 oz.)
Muffin, plain, small	1
Pancake, 4 in. across	2
Stuffing, bread (prepared)	1/4 cup
Taco shell, 6 in. across	2
Waffle, 4 1/2 in. square	1
Whole wheat crackers, fat added (such as Triscuits®)	4-6 (1 oz.)

✍ *3 grams or more of fiber per serving*

2
Meat List

Each serving of meat and substitutes on this list contains about 7 grams of protein. The amount of fat and number of calories varies, depending on what kind of meat or substitute you choose. The list is divided into three parts based on the amount of fat and calories: lean meat, medium-fat meat, and high-fat meat. One ounce (one meat exchange) of each of these includes:

	Carbohydrate (grams)	Protein (grams)	Fat (grams)	Calories
Lean	0	7	3	55
Medium-Fat	0	7	5	75
High-Fat	0	7	8	100

You are encouraged to use more lean and medium-fat meat, poultry, and fish in your meal plan. This will help decrease your fat intake, which may help decrease your risk for heart disease. The items from the high-fat group are high in saturated fat, cholesterol, and calories. You should limit your choices from the high-fat group to three (3) times per week. Meat and substitutes do not contribute any fiber to your meal plan.

TIPS

1. Bake, roast, broil, grill, or boil these foods rather than frying them with added fat.

2. Use a nonstick pan spray or a nonstick pan to brown or fry these foods.

3. Trim off visible fat before and after cooking.

4. Do not add flour, bread crumbs, coating mixes, or fat to these foods when preparing them.

5. Weigh meat after removing bones and fat, and after cooking. Three ounces of cooked meat is about equal to 4 ounces of raw meat. Some examples of meat portions are:

2 ounces meat (2 meat exchanges) =
1 small chicken leg or thigh
½ cup cottage cheese or tuna

3 ounces meat (3 meat exchanges) =
1 medium pork chop
1 small hamburger
½ of a whole chicken breast
1 unbreaded fish fillet
cooked meat about the size of a deck of cards

6. Restaurants usually serve prime cuts of meat, which are high in fat and calories.

Meats and meat substitutes that have 400 milligrams or more of sodium per exchange are indicated with this symbol.

LEAN MEAT AND SUBSTITUTES
(One exchange is equal to any one of the following items.)

Beef: USDA Good or Choice grades of lean beef, such as round, sirloin, and flank steak; tenderloin; and chipped beef ⬤   1 oz.

Pork: Lean pork, such as fresh ham; canned, cured or boiled ham ⬤; Canadian bacon ⬤, tenderloin.   1 oz.

Veal: All cuts are lean except for veal cutlets (ground or cubed). Examples of lean veal are chops and roasts.   1 oz.

Poultry: Chicken, turkey, Cornish hen (without skin)   1 oz.

Fish: All fresh and frozen fish   1 oz.
Crab, lobster, scallops, shrimp, clams (fresh or canned in water ⬤)   2 oz.
Oysters   6 medium
Tuna ⬤ (canned in water)   1/4 cup
Herring (uncreamed or smoked)   1 oz.
Sardines (canned)   2 medium

Wild Game: Venison, rabbit, squirrel   1 oz.
Pheasant, duck, goose (without skin)   1 oz.

Cheese:	Any cottage cheese	1/4 cup
	Grated parmesan	2 Tbsp.
	Diet cheeses 🔲 (with less than 55 calories per ounce)	1 oz.
Other:	95% fat-free luncheon meat	1 oz.
	Egg whites	3 whites
	Egg substitutes with less than 55 calories per 1/4 cup	1/4 cup

MEDIUM-FAT MEAT AND SUBSTITUTES
(One exchange is equal to any one of the following items.)

Beef:	Most beef products fall into this category. Examples are: all ground beef, roast (rib, chuck, rump), steak (cubed, Porterhouse, T-bone), and meatloaf.	1 oz.
Pork:	Most pork products fall into this category. Examples are: chops, loin roast, Boston butt, cutlets.	1 oz.
Lamb:	Most lamb products fall into this category. Examples are: chops, leg, and roast.	1 oz.
Veal:	Cutlet (ground or cubed, unbreaded)	1 oz.
Poultry:	Chicken (with skin), domestic duck or goose (well-drained of fat), ground turkey	1 oz.
Fish:	Tuna 🔲 (canned in oil and drained)	1/4 cup
	Salmon 🔲 (canned)	1/4 cup
Cheese:	Skim or part-skim milk cheeses, such as:	
	Ricotta	1/4 cup
	Mozzarella	1 oz.
	Diet cheeses 🔲 (with 56-80 calories per ounce)	1 oz.
Other:	86% fat-free luncheon meat 🔲	1 oz.
	Egg (high in cholesterol, limit to 3 per week)	1
	Egg substitutes with 56-80 calories per 1/4 cup	1/4 cup
	Tofu (2 1/2 in. x 2 3/4 in. x 1 in.)	4 oz.
	Liver, heart, kidney, sweetbreads	1 oz.
	(high in cholesterol)	

HIGH-FAT MEAT AND SUBSTITUTES
Remember, these items are high in saturated fat, cholesterol, and calories, and should be used only three (3) times per week.
(One exchange is equal to any one of the following items.)

Beef:	Most USDA Prime cuts of beef, such as ribs, corned beef 🔲	1 oz.
Pork:	Spareribs, ground pork, pork sausage 🔲 (patty or link)	1 oz.
Lamb:	Patties (ground lamb)	1 oz.
Fish:	Any fried fish product	1 oz.
Cheese:	All regular cheeses 🔲 , such as American, Blue, Cheddar, Monterey, Swiss	1 oz.
Other:	Luncheon meat 🔲 , such as bologna, salami, pimento loaf	1 oz.
	Sausage 🔲 , such as Polish, Italian	1 oz.
	Knockwurst, smoked	1 oz.
	Bratwurst 🔲	1 oz.
	Frankfurter 🔲 (turkey or chicken)	1 frank (10/lb.)
	Peanut butter (contains unsaturated fat)	1 Tbsp.

Count as one high-fat meat plus one fat exchange:

Frankfurter 🔲 (beef, pork, or combination)	1 frank (10/lb.)

🔲 *400 mg or more of sodium per exchange*

3
Vegetable List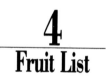

Each vegetable serving on this list contains about 5 grams of carbohydrate, 2 grams of protein, and 25 calories. Vegetables contain 2-3 grams of dietary fiber. Vegetables which contain 400 mg of sodium per serving are identified with a 🔫 symbol.

Vegetables are a good source of vitamins and minerals. Fresh and frozen vegetables have more vitamins and less added salt. Rinsing canned vegetables will remove much of the salt.

Unless otherwise noted, the serving size for vegetables (one vegetable exchange) is:

1/2 cup of cooked vegetables or vegetable juice
1 cup of raw vegetables

Artichoke (1/2 medium)
Asparagus
Beans (green, wax, Italian)
Bean sprouts
Beets
Broccoli
Brussels sprouts
Cabbage, cooked
Carrots

Cauliflower
Eggplant
Greens (collard, mustard, turnip)
Kohlrabi
Leeks
Mushrooms, cooked
Okra
Onions
Pea pods
Peppers (green)

Rutabaga
Sauerkraut 🔫
Spinach, cooked
Summer squash (crookneck)
Tomato (one large)

Tomato/vegetable juice 🔫
Turnips
Water chestnuts
Zucchini, cooked

Starchy vegetables such as corn, peas, and potatoes are found on the Starch/Bread List.

4
Fruit List

Each item on this list contains about 15 grams of carbohydrate, and 60 calories. Fresh, frozen, and dry fruits have about 2 grams of fiber per serving. Fruits that have 3 or more grams of fiber per serving have a 🥬 symbol. Fruit juices contain very little dietary fiber.

The carbohydrate and calorie content for a fruit serving are based on the usual serving of the most commonly eaten fruits. Use fresh fruits or fruits frozen or canned without sugar added. Whole fruit is more filling than fruit juice and may be a better choice for those who are trying to lose weight. Unless otherwise noted, the serving size for one fruit serving is:

1/2 cup of fresh fruit or fruit juice
1/4 cup of dried fruit

FRESH, FROZEN, AND UNSWEETENED CANNED FRUIT

Apple (raw, 2 in. across)	1 apple
Applesauce (unsweetened)	1/2 cup
Apricots (medium, raw) or	4 apricots
Apricots (canned)	1/2 cup, or 4 halves
Banana (9 in. long)	1/2 banana
🥬 Blackberries (raw)	3/4 cup
🥬 Blueberries (raw)	3/4 cup
Cantaloupe (5 in. across) (cubes)	1/3 melon 1 cup
Cherries (large, raw)	12 cherries
Cherries (canned)	1/2 cup
Figs (raw, 2 in. across)	2 figs
Fruit cocktail (canned)	1/2 cup
Grapefruit (medium)	1/2 grapefruit
Grapefruit (segments)	3/4 cup
Grapes (small)	15 grapes

Honeydew melon (medium) (cubes)	1/8 melon 1 cup
Kiwi (large)	1 kiwi
Mandarin oranges	3/4 cup
Mango (small)	1/2 mango
🥬 Nectarine (1 1/2 in. across)	1 nectarine
Orange (2 1/2 in. across)	1 orange
Papaya	1 cup
Peach (2 3/4 in. across)	1 peach, or 3/4 cup
Peaches (canned)	1/2 cup, or 2 halves
Pear	1/2 large, or 1 small
Pears (canned)	1/2 cup or 2 halves
Persimmon (medium, native)	2 persimmons
Pineapple (raw)	3/4 cup

🔫 *400 mg or more of sodium per exchange*

🥬 *3 or more grams of fiber per serving*

Pineapple (canned)	1/3 cup	
Plum (raw, 2 in. across)	2 plums	
☞ Pomegranate	1/2 pomegranate	
☞ Raspberries (raw)	1 cup	
☞ Strawberries (raw, whole)	1 1/4 cup	
Tangerine (2 1/2 in. across)	2 tangerines	
Watermelon (cubes)	1 1/4 cup	

DRIED FRUIT

☞ Apples	4 rings
☞ Apricots	7 halves
Dates	2 1/2 medium
☞ Figs	1 1/2
☞ Prunes	3 medium
Raisins	2 Tbsp.

FRUIT JUICE

Apple juice/cider	1/2 cup
Cranberry juice cocktail	1/3 cup
Grapefruit juice	1/2 cup
Grape juice	1/3 cup
Orange juice	1/2 cup
Pineapple juice	1/2 cup
Prune juice	1/3 cup

5
Milk List

Each serving of milk or milk products on this list contains about 12 grams of carbohydrate and 8 grams of protein. The amount of fat in milk is measured in percent (%) of butterfat. The calories vary, depending on what kind of milk you choose. The list is divided into three parts based on the amount of fat and calories: skim/very lowfat milk, lowfat milk, and whole milk. One serving (one milk exchange) of each of these includes:

	Carbohydrate (grams)	Protein (grams)	Fat (grams)	Calories
Skim/Very Lowfat	12	8	trace	90
Lowfat	12	8	5	120
Whole	12	8	8	150

Milk is the body's main source of calcium, the mineral needed for growth and repair of bones. Yogurt is also a good source of calcium. Yogurt and many dry or powdered milk products have different amounts of fat. If you have questions about a particular item, read the label to find out the fat and calorie content.

Milk is good to drink, but it can also be added to cereal, and to other foods. Many tasty dishes such as sugar-free pudding are made with milk.

SKIM AND VERY LOWFAT MILK

skim milk	1 cup
1/2% milk	1 cup
1% milk	1 cup
lowfat buttermilk	1 cup
evaporated skim milk	1/2 cup
dry nonfat milk	1/3 cup
plain nonfat yogurt	8 oz.

LOWFAT MILK

2% milk	1 cup fluid
plain lowfat yogurt (with added nonfat milk solids)	8 oz.

WHOLE MILK

The whole milk group has much more fat per serving than the skim and lowfat groups. Whole milk has more than 3 1/4% butterfat. Try to limit your choices from the whole milk group as much as possible.

whole milk	1 cup
evaporated whole milk	1/2 cup
whole plain yogurt	8 oz.

☞ 3 or more grams of fiber per serving

6
Fat List

Each serving on the fat list contains about 5 grams of fat and 45 calories.

The foods on the fat list contain mostly fat, although some items may also contain a small amount of protein. All fats are high in calories and should be carefully measured. Everyone should modify fat intake by eating unsaturated fats instead of saturated fats. The sodium content of these foods varies widely. Check the label for sodium information.

UNSATURATED FATS

Avocado	1/8 medium
Margarine	1 tsp.
* Margarine, diet	1 Tbsp.
Mayonnaise	1 tsp.
* Mayonnaise, reduced-calorie	1 Tbsp.

Nuts and Seeds:

Almonds, dry roasted	6 whole
Cashews, dry roasted	1 Tbsp.
Pecans	2 whole
Peanuts	20 small or 10 large
Walnuts	2 whole
Other nuts	1 Tbsp.
Seeds, pine nuts, sunflower (without shells)	1 Tbsp.
Pumpkin seeds	2 tsp.

Oil (corn, cottonseed, safflower, soybean, sunflower, olive, peanut)	1 tsp.
* Olives	10 small or 5 large
Salad dressing, mayonnaise-type	2 tsp.
Salad dressing, mayonnaise-type, reduced-calorie	1 Tbsp.
* Salad dressing (all varieties)	1 Tbsp.

🍴 Salad dressing, reduced-calorie   2 Tbsp.

(Two tablespoons of low-calorie salad dressing is a free food.)

SATURATED FATS

Butter	1 tsp.
* Bacon	1 slice
Chitterlings	1/2 ounce
Coconut, shredded	2 Tbsp.
Coffee whitener, liquid	2 Tbsp.
Coffee whitener, powder	4 tsp.
Cream (light, coffee, table)	2 Tbsp.
Cream, sour	2 Tbsp.
Cream (heavy, whipping)	1 Tbsp.
Cream cheese	1 Tbsp.
* Salt pork	1/4 ounce

---

*   *If more than one or two servings are eaten, these foods have 400 mg. or more of sodium.*

🍴 *400 mg. or more of sodium per serving.*

Weight Watchers* Food Product Information

The serving sizes of foods on the WEIGHT WATCHERS Program are not identical to the serving sizes of exchanges on the Diabetic Diet. It is quite possible to convert WEIGHT WATCHERS Program equivalencies to diabetic exchanges. This should be done, however, on the advice of your physician.

Weight Watchers International

WEIGHT WATCHERS INTERNATIONAL FOOD PRODUCT INFORMATION – UNITED STATES

	Portion Size	Calories	Protein (gm)	Carbohy-drates (gm)	Fat (gm)	WEIGHT WATCHERS program equivalencies
Apple Snacks	½ oz.	50	1	13	1	1 fruit
Fruit snacks						
Cinnamon	½ oz.	50	1	13	1	1 fruit
Peach	½ oz.	50	1	13	1	1 fruit
Strawberry	½ oz.	50	1	13	1	1 fruit
Sweet'ner – Granulated						
Sugar Substitute	1 indiv. packet	3.5	0	1	0	Use in reasonable amounts.
Soft drinks						
Black Cherry	12 fl. oz.	2	0	<1	0	2 cal. Specialty Foods
Cherry Cola	12 fl. oz.	2	0	<1	0	2 cal. Specialty Foods
Chocolate	12 fl. oz.	2	0	<1	0	2 cal. Specialty Foods
Cola	12 fl. oz.	0	0	<1	0	0 cal. Specialty Foods
Crème	12 fl. oz.	2	0	<1	0	2 cal. Specialty Foods
Frosta	12 fl. oz.	4	0	1	0	4 cal. Specialty Foods
Ginger Ale	12 fl. oz.	2	0	<1	0	2 cal. Specialty Foods
Grape	12 fl. oz.	0	0	<1	0	0 cal. Specialty Foods

WEIGHT WATCHERS INTERNATIONAL – UNITED STATES *continued*

	Portion Size	Calories	Protein (gm)	Carbohydrates (gm)	Fat (gm)	WEIGHT WATCHERS program equivalencies
Lemon-Lime	12 fl. oz.	4	0	1	0	4 cal. Specialty Foods
Orange	12 fl. oz.	2	0	<1	0	2 cal. Specialty Foods
Raspberry	12 fl. oz.	2	0	<1	0	2 cal. Specialty Foods
Rootbeer	12 fl. oz.	0	0	<1	0	0 cal. Specialty Foods
Strawberry	12 fl. oz.	2	0	<1	0	2 cal. Specialty Foods

WEIGHT WATCHERS INTERNATIONAL FOOD PRODUCT INFORMATION – CANADA

	Portion Size	Calories	Protein (gm)	Carbohydrates (gm)	Fat (gm)	WEIGHT WATCHERS program equivalencies
Calorie & carbohydrate reduced fruits						
Unpeeled Apricot Halves	4 halves with 2 T. juice	42.9	0	10.5	0	1 fruit
Fruit cocktail	½ c.	42.9	0	11.9	0	1 fruit

WEIGHT WATCHERS INTERNATIONAL—CANADA *continued*

	Portion Size	Calories	Protein (gm)	Car-bohy-drates (gm)	Fat (gm)	WEIGHT WATCHERS program equivalencies
Peach halves	2 halves with 2 T. juice	41.5	0	11.5	0	1 fruit
Sliced peaches	½ c.	42.9	0	11.9	0	1 fruit
Pear halves	2 halves with 2 T. juice	44.1	0	12.3	0	1 fruit
Plain yogurt	½ c.	46	5	6.3	0.2	1 milk
Calorie reduced fruit yogurts						
Blueberry	1 container (175 gm)	88.2	6.5	15.4	0.6	¾ milk ½ fruit
Raspberry	1 container (175 gm)	90.8	6.6	15.9	0.4	¾ milk ½ fruit
Strawberry	1 container (175 gm)	90.3	6.5	15	.04	¾ milk ½ fruit
Calorie reduced fudge bar	1 bar (75 mL)	42.8	2.4	7.6	.29	¼ milk ½ fruit

WEIGHT WATCHERS INTERNATIONAL — CANADA *continued*

	Portion Size	Calories	Protein (gm)	Car-bohy-drates (gm)	Fat (gm)	WEIGHT WATCHERS program equivalencies
Calorie reduced gelatin desserts						
Cherry	½ cup	19	2	3	0	19 Cal. Specialty Foods
Lime	½ cup	19	2	3	0	19 Cal. Specialty Foods
Raspberry	½ cup	19	2	3	0	19 Cal. Specialty Foods
Strawberry	½ cup	19	2	3	0	19 Cal. Specialty Foods
Calorie reduced iced tea mix	8 fl. oz.	20	0	5	0	20 Cal. Specialty Foods
Low calorie sodas						
Cola	1 fl. oz.	.09	0	.008	0	.09 Cal. Specialty Foods
Ginger Ale	1 fl. oz.	.1	0	.02	0	.1 Cal. Specialty Foods
Lemon-Lime	1 fl. oz.	.2	0	.04	0	.2 Cal. Specialty Foods
Orange	1 fl. oz.	.2	0	.02	0	.2 Cal. Specialty Foods
Root-Beer	1 fl. oz.	.2	0	.03	0	.2 Cal. Specialty Foods
Low calorie sweetener	1 sachet	3	0	1	0	Use in reasonable amounts.

Index